AN Rh-Hr SYLLABUS

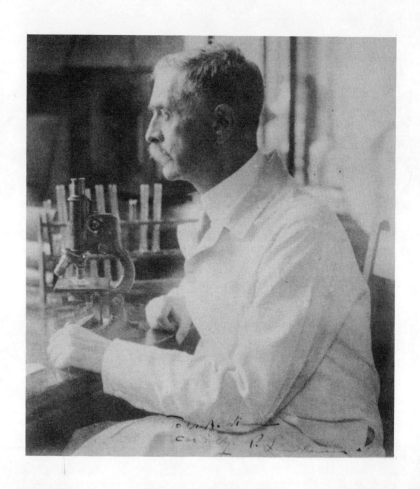

KARL LANDSTEINER
Father of Immunohematology
(1868-1943)

AN Rh-Hr SYLLABUS

The Types and Their Applications

———————————Second Edition———————————

By

ALEXANDER S. WIENER, M.D., F.A.C.P., F.C.A.P.

Associate Professor, Department of Forensic Medicine, New York University Medical School; Senior Bacteriologist (Serology) to the Office of the Chief Medical Examiner of New York City; Attending Immunohematologist, Jewish and Adelphi Hospitals, Brooklyn, N. Y.

and

IRVING B. WEXLER, M.D., F.A.A.P.

Clinical Associate Professor of Pediatrics, University of New York Downstate Medical Center; Attending Pediatrician and Associate Immunohematologist, Jewish Hospital of Brooklyn, Associate Immunohematologist, Adelphi Hospital, Brooklyn, N. Y.

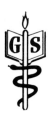

GRUNE & STRATTON • New York • 1963

Library of Congress Catalog Card No. 63-10402

Printed and bound in U.S.A. for Grune & Stratton, Inc.

B

To
Our Wives
GERTRUDE AND EDNA

Contents

Preface to the First Edition

FOLLOWING the discovery of the Rh factor with the aid of anti-rhesus immune serum in 1937, the Rh-Hr types developed into a complex subject with important applications in clinical medicine, legal medicine, and anthropology. The purpose of this booklet is to present an up-to-date summary of the subject in a compact, easily understandable form. This has been accomplished by presenting the information in the form of a glossary, arranged in logical order, so that the booklet can be read through readily from beginning to end. Though the presentation is compact and simple, an attempt has been made to be as comprehensive as possible so that no facet of the subject has been neglected. To facilitate finding answers to specific questions an index is included.

The booklet not only presents the complex serology and genetics of the Rh-Hr types, but provides brief directions for performing Rh antibody tests and titrations by the agglutination, conglutination, blocking, antiglobulin, and enzyme methods. It also presents details concerning erythroblastosis fetalis, exchange transfusion, hemolytic transfusion reactions, the racial distribution of the Rh-Hr types and their application in disputed paternity, and the interesting subject of autosensitization. In developing the complex subject of Rh-Hr genetics, only the international Rh-Hr nomenclature is used, for reasons which will become evident to the reader as he masters the subject. In brief, the letters C-D-E are even more inadequate for the Rh-Hr types than the numbers 1-2-3-4 were for the A-B-O groups.

No bibliography is given, and no attempt is made to offer a detailed analysis of the thousands of publications in the field. Those requiring a more thorough treatment of the subject are referred to a previous book of the author's, *Blood Groups and Transfusion*, for a review of the literature up to 1943, and to his recently published book, *The Rh-Hr Blood Types; Applications in Clinical and Legal Medicine and Anthropology*, for the developments during the decade 1943 to 1953. The present volume serves as a convenient introduction to the other volumes. For readers not specializing in the field, it contains all the information they require and will make it possible for them to read and understand without difficulty current articles on the subject, no matter how complex.

The author wishes to acknowledge his appreciation to Miss Nancy Ercolono for her patient and expert assistance in the preparation of this manuscript for publication, and to Mr. Henry M. Stratton for his helpful encouragement and advice.

A. S. WIENER

Brooklyn, N. Y.
September 1953

Preface to the Second Edition

SEVEN YEARS have passed since the first edition of this monograph was published. That the volume has served a useful purpose is indicated by its having been out of print for the past three years. Rather than attempt to satisfy the continuing demand by reprinting the book in its original form, it was decided to prepare a new edition, in order to include information which has come to light in the interval. For this task the senior author has enlisted the help of his associate, friend and collaborator of many years' standing, Dr. I. B. Wexler.

The plan of the first edition has been retained, namely, to present the information in the form of a glossary. In this way the presentation becomes simple, compact and as readable as possible. No bibliography is included, but the reader who is interested in having more detailed information may consult Wiener's *Blood Groups and Transfusion* for literature up to 1943, Wiener's *Rh-Hr Blood Types* for the literature covering the decade 1943 to 1953, and to Wiener and Wexler's *Heredity of the Blood Groups* and Wiener's *Advances in Blood Grouping* for the literature on the subject up to 1960.

Certain aspects of the subject were considered controversial at the time that the first edition of this syllabus was published. In the interval, additional information and evidence have accumulated so that the facts can no longer be denied. For example, a series of definitive reports on the complexities of Rh-Hr serology and nomenclature has been published by the Committee on Medicolegal Problems of the American Medical Association. That committee has recommended that the Rh-Hr terminology be adopted exclusively while the C-D-E notations should not be used, in conformity with the plan followed in the first edition of this syllabus. Since the evidence on which this decision is based is given in detail in the committee reports, which can be obtained by writing to the Law Department of the American Medical Association, 535 North Dearborn Street, Chicago 10, Ill., no space will be devoted to the subject of nomenclature here. It is recognized that a large segment of workers in the field continue to use the C-D-E notations. The present authors, however, find the C-D-E symbols cumbersome and inadequate for presenting the latest discoveries in the field. Moreover, it is not possible to translate from one nomenclature to the other, except in the simplest situations, because the C-D-E notations misrepresent the facts observed in the laboratory and have been responsible for numerous fallacies that have appeared in the literature. Readers who would like a detailed explanation and discussion of this subject may consult the present authors' 1958 book, *The Heredity of the Blood Groups*, as well as Wiener's *Advances in Blood Grouping*, which appeared in 1961.

An important feature of the Rh-Hr nomenclature is the use of symbols printed in special type to represent different things and ideas. As in the former edition of this syllabus, regular type is used for agglutinogens, phenotypes and blood group systems, as well as for general statements, while **bold-faced** type is used for symbols representing blood factors and their corresponding specific antibodies. *Italics* are used for the symbols for genes and genotypes.

While an Rh-Hr syllabus must include all aspects of serology and genetics, including the most esoteric, if it is to satisfy all the needs of workers in the field, the general reader requires simple statements of the basic facts and simplified explanations of their applications in clinical medicine. This the syllabus also attempts to provide. The general reader may skip those portions of the syllabus which do not interest him, and quickly find the information he requires with the aid of the index and the table of contents. The book may also prove useful for the specialist in forensic medicine who is interested in the medicolegal applications of blood grouping, as well as to the physical anthropologist and the veterinarian.

It is hoped that this second edition will be well received, and the authors would appreciate any criticisms and suggestions from readers which may prove helpful in the preparation of future editions.

The preparation of this new edition was aided in part by grant RG 9237, U.S.P.H.S. The authors are also indebted to their good friend and publisher, Dr. Henry Stratton, for his encouragement and advice in the preparation of this monograph.

Brooklyn, New York   A. S. WIENER
                                                          I. B. WEXLER

CHAPTER I

Fundamentals

Antigen: Any substance which when introduced into the body, usually by a parenteral route, stimulates the production of specifically reacting substances. Antigens are usually foreign to the body and are not necessarily toxic or pathogenic. They may be soluble substances such as toxins and foreign proteins, or particulate, such as bacteria or tissue cells. The antigens with which this book is primarily concerned are red blood cells.

Antibodies: Specifically reacting substances produced by the body in response to the introduction of antigen. The best evidence available indicates that antibodies are produced by plasma cells at the germinal centers of the lymph nodes, and occur in the plasma as modified serum gamma globulins. Antibodies differ from normal serum gamma globulin molecules in that a portion of the surface (the "active patch") has been modified to become a counterpart of the antigen. That the active patch makes up only a relatively small fraction of the antibody molecule seems evident, since antibodies and normal serum globulin are indistinguishable except for the ability of the former to combine with their corresponding antigens.

Specificity: One of the most important attributes of antibodies and their reactions. The specificity of antigen-antibody reactions is in many ways comparable to the specificity of a key for a particular lock. Thus, the specificity of antibodies is not absolute, but may extend to substances of related chemical structure, just as keys can open more than one lock. Reactions of antibodies with antigens other than those that caused their formation are called cross reactions. All antibodies have both specific and cross-reacting characteristics.

Agglutinogen: A substance on the surface of cells (red cells and bacteria), so named because when combined with a corresponding antibody, clumping (or agglutination) of the cells results. Since combination of agglutinogen and antibody in the presence of complement may lead to lysis, the name agglutinogen is not always appro-

1

priate, but is nonetheless convenient. (The term "phenogroup" has been applied for the corresponding substances on the red cells of cattle, because hemolytic tests are used exclusively in those animals.) For red cells the more complete name hemagglutinogen is sometimes used.

Agglutinin: The name applied to antibodies demonstrable by agglutination tests. The term hemolysin is used when the antibody produces lysis. To produce lysis the presence of complement is essential. While alpha and beta antibodies (of the A-B-O groups) can produce both hemolysis and agglutination under appropriate conditions, specific hemolysis does not occur in the Rh-Hr tests.

Complement: A thermolabile complex of proteins in normal blood serum which causes lysis of bacteria or red cells which have combined with their specific antibodies. Instead of hemolysin the antibody is often called amboceptor in conformity with Ehrlich's concept of an antibody having two receptors, one combining with the cells and the other with complement.

Isoantibody: An antibody which reacts with antigens from animals in the same species; e.g., the Rh-Hr antibodies discussed in this book are isoantibodies.

Heteroantibody: An antibody which reacts with antigens derived from animals of a different species; e.g., the original anti-rhesus serum produced by Landsteiner and Wiener by immunizing rabbits and guinea pigs contained heteroantibodies for human as well as rhesus red cells.

Autoantibody: Antibodies reactive with antigens present in the same animal; e.g., the antibodies for acquired autohemolytic anemia and those found in disseminated lupus erythematosus are autoantibodies.

Serological factor: One of the multiple serological specificities of an antigenic substance. An antigenic substance which has the capacity to react with an antibody to which has been assigned the symbol anti-**X** is said to have the serologic factor **X**. To distinguish clearly between symbols for antigenic substances and their serologic factors, regular type is used for the former and bold face for the latter. Bold face is therefore also necessarily used for the corresponding antibody symbol.

Cross-reactivity: The capacity of antibodies to react not only with their homologous antigen, but also with other antigens. As is to be expected, cross reactions occur with antigens of related structure, since chemical composition is the ultimate basis for antigen-antibody specificity. Thus, antibodies against red cells of one species generally cross-react with red cells of a related species; e.g., anti-horse with donkey, anti-human with chimpanzee, etc. The ability of two antigenic substances to react with the same antibody does not imply necessarily the presence of identical chemical structures, or even identical groupings. Mere similarity of the surface structure is sufficient. Therefore, theoretically, every antibody can react with an unlimited number of different antigens.

Heterogenetic antibodies: Antibodies that cross-react with antigens apparently unrelated to the antigen which stimulated their production. The classic heterogenetic antibodies are the Frossman antibodies, exemplified by the immune sera for guinea pig kidney which lyse sheep red cells. Similarly, the Paul-Bunnell test used for the diagnosis of infectious mononucleosis depends on a heterogenetic antibody, since sheep cells obviously have no bearing on the pathogenesis of the disease; the Wassermann antibody (for beef heart antigen) is likewise of heterogenetic origin. Schiff and Adelsberger showed that rabbit immune sera for group A blood may hemolyze sheep blood cells in high dilutions, and conversely anti-sheep immune rabbit sera may have blood group A specificity. Similarly, the Rh blood factor of human blood was discovered with the aid of a heterogenetic immune rabbit serum for blood from M. rhesus monkeys, as indicated by its symbol Rh (for rhesus).

Heterogenetic antibodies may be compared to skeleton keys, and their cross reactions have been ascribed to similarities in the surface structure of the antigen molecules. They provide a striking example of the capacity of antibodies in general to cross-react (*cf.* fig. 1).

Combining groups: The sites on the surface of the antigen molecule with which the antibody combines. Different antibodies may have different combining sites, but the combining sites for different antibodies may also overlap as shown in figure 1. Therefore, theoretically, each antigenic substance or even each combining group of the antigenic substance may elicit the formation of an unlimited number of different specific antibodies. Moreover, just as every

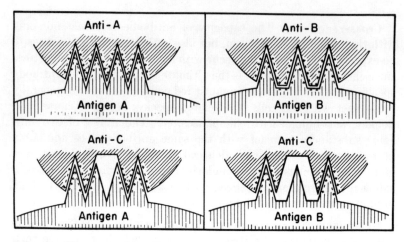

Fig. 1.—Diagrammatic representation of the nature of cross reactions. The letters **A**, **B**, and **C** have no reference to the A-B-O blood groups, but are used to designate any hypothetic serologic factors. (Wiener, A. S., and Wexler, I. B.: Bact. Rev. *16:* 69, 1952.)

antibody can theoretically combine with an unlimited number of different antigens, so every antigen can combine with an unlimited number of different antibodies.

Blood factor: The serologic factors of red cell agglutinogens are called blood factors. Red cell agglutinogens are characterized by multiple blood factors. For example, agglutinogen A has in addition to blood factor **A** the factor F_A which is shared with sheep cells (mentioned under Heterogenetic antibodies) and factor **C** which it shares with agglutinogen B. Agglutinogens are named after the most important blood factor or factors that characterize them; e.g., agglutinogen A is so named after its blood factor **A**; the less important factors F_A and **C** being omitted from the name. It is evident that the complete serological identification of an antigen does not depend upon tests with merely a single antiserum (for a single blood factor), but on multiple tests with different antisera to identify the *set* of blood factors characteristic of the agglutinogen.

Blood grouping: Classification of blood specimens into groups (or types) on the basis of the blood factors or agglutinogens which they contain.

Blood group system: A system of related blood factors and agglutinogens, e.g., the A-B-O system, the M-N-S system, the Rh-Hr

system, etc. The relationship between the blood factors and agglutinogens to form a system is established by studying the distribution
in the population, and by heredity studies on families.

There is evidence that the agglutinogens are arranged more or less
regularly on the surface of the erythrocyte, there being separate
locations or loci for each blood group system (*cf.* fig. 2). Apparently
the A-B-O agglutinogens are far more numerous than the Rh-Hr
agglutinogens, which in turn appear to be more numerous than the
K (or Kell) and F (or Duffy) agglutinogens.

Normal or natural antibodies: Antibodies occurring in serum
without any apparent antigenic stimulus, in contrast to immune

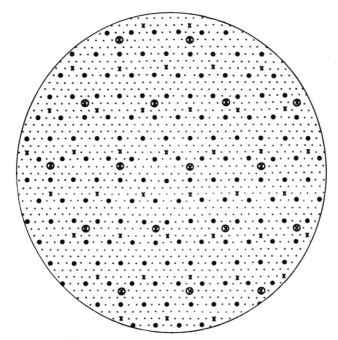

●- A-B-O Haptenes
✗- M-N Haptenes
⊕- Rh-Hr Haptenes
•- Haptenes of other specificities ; species specific

Fig. 2.—Diagrammatic representation of the hypothetical
arrangement of agglutinogens about the periphery of the human
erythrocyte.

antibodies. It is probable that most if not all so-called normal antibodies are of immune origin, since they occur under circumstances in which inapparent infections cannot be ruled out. Similarly, normally occurring hemagglutinins such as anti-**A** and anti-**B** and the cold autoantibodies are also probably of heterogenetic immune origin, due to inapparent infections with microorganisms possessing antigens chemically related to the blood group mucopolysaccharides (*cf*. "Heterogenetic antibodies" on page 3). Natural antibodies can be compared to skeleton keys and are poorly adapted or low avidity antibodies. Characteristically, therefore, natural hemagglutinins give their strongest reactions at low (refrigerator) temperature, since at higher (body) temperature thermal agitation tends to disrupt the weakly bound antigen-antibody complex. Natural antibodies for the Rh factor are extremely rare, if they occur at all, in contrast to anti-**A** and anti-**B**, which, after the first year of life, are regularly present in the serum whenever the corresponding blood factor **A** or **B** is absent from the cells (Landsteiner's rule).

Immunization; sensitization: The process whereby the body is stimulated to produce specific antibodies. This may occur spontaneously, as during the course of an infection, the antigen in that case being the invading microorganism. Experimentally, as for the production of typing serum, the antigen is introduced parenterally, generally by the intravenous route.

Immunologic paralysis: A phenomenon in which the body has lost its capacity to respond to a particular antigen. This was first described by Felton, who attributed it to the flooding of the body with massive doses of the antigen. This appears to interfere with the capacity to produce specific antibodies, though not to unrelated antigens. It is probably identical with the phenomenon named immunologic tolerance by more recent workers, and is also probably related to, if not identical with, the phenomenon called *horror autotoxicus* by Ehrlich, and the self-marker hypothesis of Burnet.

Anti-rhesus serum: In the narrow sense, antiserum prepared in rabbits, guinea pigs, goats, and other animals by injections of blood of rhesus monkeys. Thus, the term applies to the original experimental sera of Landsteiner and Wiener, which clump the bloods of 85 per cent of Caucasoids. In the broad sense, the term has been applied to include all the related Rh-Hr antisera of human origin.

Isosensitization; isoimmunization: Production of group specific isoantibodies by an individual of a species as a result of the injection of blood from a different member of the same species, as contrasted to heteroimmunization with blood or organs of a foreign species, and autoimmunization or immunization against substances present in the individual's own body. Rh antibodies are produced by Rh-negative human beings by isoimmunization, either as a result of a transfusion or an intramuscular injection of Rh-positive blood, or pregnancy with an Rh-positive fetus.

Rhesus factors; Rh factors: The factors of human blood upon which the specific combination with rhesus antibodies depend. Study of anti-Rh sera of human origin show that there exist in human blood a variety of blood factors related to the original rhesus factor of Landsteiner and Wiener, and the terms rhesus factors or Rh factors are often used to include all of these related blood factors of the Rh-Hr system. Of the various rhesus factors, the one corresponding to the original factor is designated **Rh$_0$**. The rhesus factors are divided into two subclasses of related factors; those factors more closely related to the original rhesus factor are called Rh factors, while certain reciprocally related factors are called Hr factors, in conformity with Levine's suggestion. A list of the most important Rh-Hr factors, the existence of which has been established, is shown in table 1. As has already been pointed out, the number of Rh-Hr factors theoretically possible is unlimited. For this reason, the exact specificities of antibodies still to be discovered is largely unpredictable.

Specificity: This was defined by Karl Landsteiner as disproportional reactivity. If, as shown in table 2a, in direct tests with antisera arbitrarily designated as anti-**X** and anti-**Y**, antigenic substance A reacts with anti-**X** but not with anti-**Y**, while substance B reacts with anti-**Y** and not with anti-**X**, clearly two different specificities are being detected. On the other hand, if in tests on a series of bloods, two antisera anti-**S** and anti-**T** always give parallel reactions, presumably they are identical. If, however, there are some bloods, S− T+, but none S+ T−, the two sera may have different specificities, or one may merely be weaker than the other. Which is the correct explanation can be determined by titration, as shown in table 2b.

TABLE 1.—*List of Known Rh-Hr Antibodies and Blood Factors*

Antibodies	Blood Factors	Antibodies	Blood Factors
1. $\begin{cases} \text{Anti-rhesus} \\ \text{Anti-}\mathbf{Rh_0} \end{cases}$	$\mathbf{Rh_0}$ and $\mathfrak{Rh_0}$	10. Anti-$\mathbf{rh^{w2}}$	$\mathbf{rh^{w2}}$
		11. Anti-$\mathbf{rh^{G}}$	$\mathbf{rh^{G}}$
2. Anti-$\mathbf{rh'}$	$\mathbf{rh'}$	12. Anti-$\mathbf{rh_i}$	$\mathbf{rh_i}$
3. Anti-$\mathbf{hr'}$	$\mathbf{hr'}$	13. Anti-$\mathbf{Rh^A}$	$\mathbf{Rh^A}$
4. Anti-$\mathbf{rh''}$	$\mathbf{rh''}$	14. Anti-$\mathbf{Rh^B}$	$\mathbf{Rh^B}$
5. Anti-$\mathbf{hr''}$	$\mathbf{hr''}$	15. Anti-$\mathbf{Rh^C}$	$\mathbf{Rh^C}$
6. *Anti-$\mathbf{rh^{w1}}$	$\mathbf{rh^{w1}}$	16. Anti-$\mathbf{Rh^D}$	$\mathbf{Rh^D}$
7. Anti-$\mathbf{hr}$	$\mathbf{hr}$	17. Anti-$\mathbf{Hr}$	$\mathbf{Hr}$
8. Anti-$\mathbf{rh^X}$	$\mathbf{rh^X}$	18. Anti-$\mathbf{hr^S}$	$\mathbf{hr^S}$
9. Anti-$\mathbf{hr^V}$	$\mathbf{hr^V}$		

The blood factors have been arranged chronologically in the order of their discovery.

* When symbol $\mathbf{rh^w}$ is used, this refers to factor $\mathbf{rh^w}$ and not to $\mathbf{rh^{w2}}$.

TABLE 2.—*Hypothetical Reactions Illustrating the Nature of Serological Specificity*

a. Tests by Direct Reaction

Antigenic substances	Antisera detecting different serologic specificities		Antisera which may or may not be detecting different specificities	
	Anti-X	Anti-Y	Anti-S	Anti-T
A	+	−	−	+
B	−	+	+	+

b. Tests by Titration

Antigenic substances	Antisera showing disproportional reactivity, and therefore differences in specificity		Antisera showing proportional reactivity, and therefore presumably of the same specificity	
	Anti-X	Anti-Y	Anti-S	Anti-T
A	500	50	10	100
B	1000	1000	0	5
C	0	25	500	5000

Rhesus antibodies; Rh antibodies: The anti-rhesus (anti-Rh) sera prepared by immunizing animals with rhesus monkey blood cells give reactions in tests on human red cells parallel with those observed using human antisera of the specificity designated anti-Rh_0. Of the anti-rhesus (anti-Rh) antibodies in human serum which are listed in table 1, the seven most often used in diagnostic tests are the following: Rh antibodies: anti-Rh_0, anti-rh′, anti-rh″ and anti-rh^w; Hr antibodies: anti-hr′, anti-hr″, and anti-hr.

When a serum containing an antibody belonging to the Rh-Hr system is found which gives reactions not corresponding to any of the previously described antibodies, an appropriate new symbol must be coined. Before this is done, comparative tests must be carried out with all the known antibodies, and differences in specificity shown to be present.

Rh_0 factor; standard Rh factor: The Rh blood factor corresponding to the original rhesus factor of Landsteiner and Wiener, present in blood specimens from approximately 85 per cent of Caucasians, approximately 90 per cent of Negroes, and almost 100 per cent of Mongolians. This is the most antigenic of the Rh-Hr factors, and therefore the most important clinically. Thus, sensitization to the Rh_0 factor is responsible for more than 90 per cent of the severe cases of erythroblastosis fetalis and intragroup hemolytic transfusion reactions. When the term Rh factor is used without qualification, therefore, it is the most important factor, Rh_0, which is intended.

Antigenicity: The capacity to stimulate the formation of antibodies. The factor Rh_0 is said to be the most antigenic of the Rh-Hr factors because most individuals lacking factor Rh_0 are readily sensitized by injections of Rh_0-positive blood. In contrast, individuals lacking other Rh-Hr factors are not readily sensitized by injections of blood having the missing blood factor. Of the other Rh-Hr factors, hr′ appears to be the most antigenic.

Anti-Rh_0 serum; standard anti-Rh serum: Antiserum specific for the Rh_0 blood factor. Anti-Rh_0 serum of human origin (isoimmune Rh_0 antiserum) is of greater avidity and specificity than animal immune anti-rhesus serum (heteroimmune Rh_0 antiserum). This is reasonable since the former may be compared to an exact key for a lock and the latter to a skeleton key. Moreover, anti-rhesus immune animal serum clumps all blood specimens from newborn babies, whether Rh positive or Rh negative, and more strongly than it clumps Rh-positive adult blood. Therefore, at present, only human anti-**Rh**$_0$ is used for diagnostic tests, and the original immune anti-rhesus serum is now mainly of theoretic and historical interest.

Avidity: The intensity of the affinity and union between antigen and antibody. In *in vitro* tests, this is measured by the speed with which visible clumping appears, and the size of the clumps.

Nonreciprocal reactions: Immune serum for antigen A may contain, in addition to the specific antibody anti-**A**, another antibody cross-reacting with a different antigen B; on the other hand, immune serum for antigen B may fail to cross-react with antigen A. This phenomenon was called a nonreciprocal reaction by Landsteiner. Similarly, although anti-rhesus immune rabbit and guinea-pig sera cross-react with human Rh-positive red cells, anti-**Rh**$_0$ isoimmune human serum does not cross-react with rhesus blood cells. A diagrammatic representation of nonreciprocal reactions is shown in figure 3. This is merely another aspect of the mosaic structure of agglutinogens, and demonstrates that there is more than one kind of **Rh**$_0$ factor; namely, one related to a factor present in rhesus monkey red cells, and another peculiar to human and chimpanzee blood cells alone.

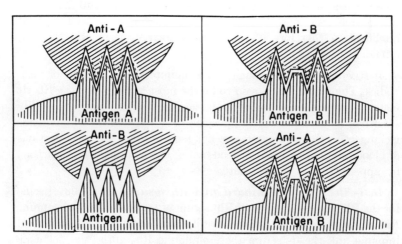

Fig. 3.—Diagrammatic representation of the nature of nonreciprocal reactions. (Wiener, A. S., and Wexler, I. B.: Bact. Rev. *16:* 69, 1952.)

Rh factors: There are three principal Rh factors: **Rh$_0$** (present in approximately 85 per cent of Caucasians), **rh′** (70 per cent positive), and **rh″** (30 per cent positive). The symbol **Rh$_0$** has a capital "R" to indicate its special serological and genetic position, while **rh′** and **rh″** have small "r's" to indicate their subordinate position. The various Rh factors do not necessarily all represent separate structures on the red cell envelope, or even different combining groups within a single molecule, but are extrinsic attributes of complex structures, the Rh agglutinogens, each of which is characterized by its own specific set of Rh factors. A fourth Rh factor, **rh^{w1}**, occurs only in association with the factor **rh′**, which is additional evidence that the factors do not necessarily represent separable structures.

Hr factors: Blood factors reciprocally related to the Rh factors. In fact, the symbol Hr was invented by Levine to indicate this relationship to Rh. To date, antisera for factor **hr′** (80 per cent positive) and **hr″** (98 per cent positive) have been found, but no reagent has been found for the theoretically possible **Hr$_0$** factor (theoretic frequency, 65 per cent). Instead, a different blood factor designated **hr** has been found (frequency 65 per cent).

Rh testing: Classifying human blood by tests with anti-**Rh$_0$** serum alone. By such tests two types only are distinguishable, namely, Rh positive and Rh negative—or, more strictly, **Rh$_0$** positive and **Rh$_0$** negative. When the terms Rh positive and Rh negative are used without qualification, it is the **Rh$_0$** factor which is intended.

Rh typing: Classification of blood into one of eight types by tests with all three standard Rh antisera; anti-**Rh$_0$**, anti-**rh′**, and anti-**rh″**. The scheme of the eight Rh types (table 3) is readily learned because of its analogy to the scheme of the four Landsteiner blood groups, after which the names of the Rh types were modeled by Wiener. Thus, there are four Rh-negative types, rh, rh′, rh″, and rh′rh″ (now named rh$_y$), and four Rh-positive types, Rh$_0$, Rh$_1$, Rh$_2$, and Rh$_1$Rh$_2$ (now named Rh$_z$). For blood transfusions to Rh-negative recipients, only type rh (triple Rh negative) donors should be used, to avoid sensitization to the **rh′** and **rh″** factors. On the other hand, recipients or expectant mothers of type rh′, rh″ or rh$_y$, as well as type rh, must be considered Rh negative, since they lack the most antigenic factor **Rh$_0$**, and therefore are likely candidates for Rh sensitization.

TABLE 3.—*Scheme of the Eight Rh Types*

Rh$_0$-negative Types				Rh$_0$-positive Types			
Designation of types	Reactions with serum			Designation of types	Reactions with serum		
	Anti-rh′	Anti-rh″	Anti-Rh$_0$		Anti-rh′	Anti-rh″	Anti-Rh$_0$
rh	−	−	−	Rh$_0$	−	−	+
rh′	+	−	−	Rh$_1$	+	−	+
rh″	−	+	−	Rh$_2$	−	+	+
rh$_y$	+	+	−	Rh$_z$	+	+	+

The types are named after the Rh blood factors (and agglutinogens) present in the red cells, Rh$_1$ being short for Rh$_0$rh′ (or Rh$_0'$) and Rh$_2$ short for Rh$_0$rh″ (or Rh$_0''$). Similarly, rh$_y$ is used in place of rh′rh″ and Rh$_z$ in place of Rh$_1$Rh$_2$ (or Rh$_0'$Rh$_0''$).

(Wiener, A. S.: Dade County M. A. Bull. *20:* 20, 1949.)

TABLE 4.—*Representative Data on the Racial Distribution of the Eight Rh Types*

Ethnic Group	Approximate Frequency (per cent) of Rh Blood Types							
	rh	rh′	rh″	rh$_y$	Rh$_0$	Rh$_1$	Rh$_2$	Rh$_z$
Caucasoids (N.Y.C.)[1]	13.5	1.0	0.5	.02	2.5	53.0	15.0	14.5
Negroids								
N.Y.C.[2]..........	7.5	1.5	0	0	45.0	25.0	15.5	5.5
Africa[3]..........	3.75	0.75	0	0	70.0	15.0	9.0	1.5
Puerto Ricans[4]......	10.1	1.7	0.5	0	15.1	39.1	19.6	14.0
Chinese[5]...........	1.5	0	0	0	0.9	60.6	3.0	34.4
Japanese[6]..........	0.6	0	0	0	0	51.7	8.3	39.4
Filipinos[7]..........	0	0	0	0	0	87.0	2.0	11.0
Mexican Indians[8]....	0	0	0	0	1.1	48.1	9.5	41.2

(Modified after Wiener, A. S.: Am. J. Clin. Path. *16:* 477, 1946).

[1] Wiener et al.; Unger et al.; Levine.
[2] Wiener et al.; Levine.
[3] Hubinont et al.
[4] Torregrosa.
[5] Wiener et al.
[6] Waller and Levine; Miller and Taguchi.
[7] Simmons and Graydon.
[8] Wiener et al.

The differences in distribution of the eight Rh types in a few representative human populations are shown in table 4. Caucasoids have the highest frequency of type rh, Mongoloids the lowest, while Negroids are characterized by a very high frequency of type Rh_0. So strikingly different are the distributions of the Rh types in these three racial groups that Rh typing has proved of great value in studies of racial crossing (compare, for example, Negroids of New York City and Africa, and Puerto Ricans, in table 4).

CHAPTER II

Rh Antibodies

Univalent antibodies: One form in which antibodies of any given specificity may occur. Univalent antibodies tend to appear later in the course of sensitization, are relatively thermostable, and readily pass through the intact placenta. Univalent Rh_0 antibodies will combine with and coat Rh-positive cells in a saline medium, but without clumping them. In protein media, or in the presence of high molecular weight colloids, univalent Rh antibodies clump cells having the corresponding specific blood factor.

Bivalent antibodies: Another form in which antibodies of a given specificity can occur. Such antibodies are usually produced early in the course of immunization, are relatively thermolabile, and are effectively held back by the intact placental barrier. In saline as well as colloidal media, they are capable of directly clumping cells possessing the corresponding specific agglutinogen.

The differences between univalent and bivalent antibodies are summarized more fully in table 5. It must be borne in mind that while the concept of difference of valence is helpful when visualizing the *in vitro* reactions of Rh agglutinating and Rh blocking sera (*cf.* figs. 4 and 5), it is possible to explain the reactions in other ways; for example, on the basis of the difference in molecular size alone. Therefore, the concept of valence is not to be taken too literally, and "univalent" antibody and "bivalent" antibody should be considered merely convenient names for distinguishing the two major forms in which antibodies of a single specificity can occur.

Agglutination: Specific clumping of cells produced by bivalent antibodies.

Conglutination: Specific clumping of cells by the combined action of univalent antibodies and conglutinin. Conglutination, as originally defined, requires in addition to the antibody the presence of a thermolabile non-specific component related to or identical with

TABLE 5.—*Properties of Univalent and Bivalent Antibodies*

Characteristic	Bivalent Antibodies	Univalent Antibodies
Common names	Agglutinin, precipitin, agglutinating antibody, complete antibody	Glutinin, blocking antibody, conglutinating antibody, incomplete antibody
Usual time of appearance in course of immunization	Early	Late
Resistance to heating	Relatively thermolabile	Relatively thermostable
Reactions of Rh-Hr antibodies* in saline medium	Clumps cells by agglutination	Coats cells without clumping them—blocking reaction
Reactions of Rh-Hr antibodies in colloid medium	Clumps cells by agglutination	Clumps cells by conglutination
Reaction in presence of complement	Does not fix complement or lyse cells	Fixes complement and lyses cells if the number of antigenic loci on cells surface is adequate; viz., lysis occurs in A-B-O and Vel tests but not in Rh-Hr, Kell, or Duffy tests.
Behavior in mixed agglutination tests	Specific clumps are formed	Clumps contain more than than one kind of cell
Opsonic effect	None	Positive in presence of complement
Chemical nature	Euglobulin; precipitated by sodium sulphate solutions of concentrations 13.5 to 17.4 per cent	Pseudoglobulin; precipitated by sodium sulphate solutions of concentrations 17.4 to 21.5 per cent
Electrophoretic behavior	Beta and gamma globulins	Gamma globulins
Sedimentation constant	19S	7S
Probable molecular weight	930,000	155,000
Diffusibility	Poor	Good
Behavior relative to placenta	Held back by intact placenta	Passes through placenta readily
Half-life	Probably 2 weeks or less	30 to 35 days
Role in syphilis	Flocculating antibody	Complement fixing antibody
Role in disease	Precipitating and agglutinating antibody	Protective antibody; antitoxin
Role in allergy	Sensitizing antibody (reagin)	Blocking antibody
Role in erythroblastosis	Not significant	Major
Role in blood transfusion	Important	Important

* The in vitro reactions are somewhat different, depending on the antigen-antibody system.

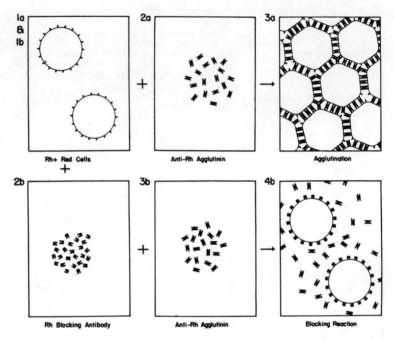

FIG. 4.—Diagrammatic visualization of the Rh agglutination and blocking reactions. Tests in saline mediums. (Wiener, A. S.: Am. J. Clin. Path. *16:* 477, 1946.)

complement. In the conglutination tests carried out with Rh-Hr antibodies, however, the presence of complement is not required.

Conglutinin: A colloidal aggregate of serum proteins which, when adsorbed by cells which have been sensitized (or coated) by their specific univalent antibodies, causes them to stick together (conglutination). Conglutinin is related to complement but is relatively thermostable. When conglutinin is diluted with crystalline solutions, it is inactivated, apparently due to dissociation of the complex into its constituent molecules. The concentration of conglutinin in the serum of fetuses and newborn infants is less than that in adult serum, paralleling the lower protein content of the former.

Conglutinin substitutes: Surface colloids of complex molecular structure, such as acacia, gelatin, dextran, and PVP, which may take the place of plasma in the conglutination test. Their ability to

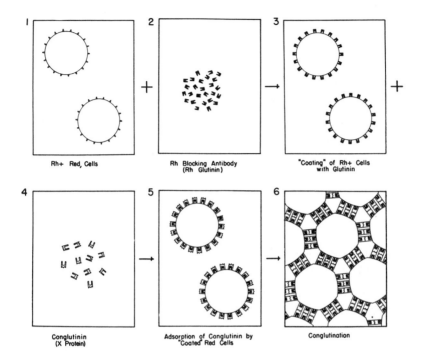

FIG. 5.—Diagrammatic visualization of the Rh conglutination reaction. Tests in plasma or colloid mediums. (Wiener, A. S.: Am. J. Clin. Path. *16:* 477, 1946.)

produce conglutination is due to their cohesive and adhesive properties, but they have the disadvantage of causing cells to clump weakly even when they are not coated or sensitized by univalent antibody, an undesirable property which makes these substances unsuitable for Rh tests, because of the danger of non-specific reactions.

Fortified conglutinin: Conglutinin which has been improved by the addition of optimal amounts of albumin. For example, it has been found that when oxalated plasma is mixed with one-fourth its volume of 30 per cent bovine albumin (Armour), its conglutinating activity is considerably enhanced.

Rh antisera, anti-Rh sera: anti-rhesus sera: Sera of human origin containing Rh and/or Hr antibodies. The antibodies in such sera may occur singly, as in sera of specificity anti-Rh_0, anti-rh', anti-**rh**″, anti-**rh**ᵂ¹, anti-**hr**′, anti-**hr**″, and anti-**hr**, or in combinations, such as the polyvalent sera anti-**Rh**$_0$′, anti-**Rh**$_0$″, anti-**rh**″**hr**′, and anti-**rh**′**hr**″. These antisera are generally obtained from patients who have had hemolytic transfusion reactions or who have given birth to erythroblastotic babies. Only sera containing antibodies of high titer and avidity are suitable for use as diagnostic reagents.

Rh agglutinating serum: Serum containing Rh antibodies predominantly of the bivalent variety. Such antisera usually give best results by the tube agglutination method, in which one drop of a 2 per cent saline suspension of red cells and a drop of testing serum are mixed in a small test tube, and the reactions read after incubation for 60 to 120 minutes at body temperature. Such reactions can often be improved by light centrifugation (500 rpm) for 1 minute. With satisfactory antisera the reactions are very sharp, but the clumps are much more fragile than those obtained in A-B-O grouping, so that the tubes must be handled gently.

Rh conglutinating serum: Serum containing Rh antibodies predominantly of the univalent variety. Such sera give good results by a variety of techniques utilizing the principle of conglutination. For example, in the slide method, a drop of antiserum is mixed with one or two drops of the whole, undiluted oxalated blood being tested on a warmed open slide, the mixture is spread over an area about an inch in diameter, and the reactions read with the naked eye after the slide has been tilted back and forth for a minute or two over a warmed viewing box. Tube techniques may also be used; for example, by using cell suspensions diluted with plasma or albumin, instead of saline solution.

It is important to bear in mind that all Rh antisera probably contain a mixture of both the univalent and the bivalent forms of antibodies. Where the univalent antibodies predominate, the antisera may be used by a conglutination method; where bivalent antibodies predominate, the tube agglutination method may be used. When antiserum containing a suitable balanced mixture of **Rh**$_0$ agglutinating and blocking antibodies is titrated in saline medium, a prozone may occur. In the so-called rapid tube conglutination test, two drops of antiserum are placed in a tube and, by using a wooden applicator, enough red cells are carried over into the tube from the blood clot to make a 2 to 4 per cent suspension in the serum. This mixture is centrifuged briefly and the sediment resuspended by gentle shaking before the reactions are read. The antisera used in this test are fortified by the addition of bovine albumin by the manufacturers before distribution.

Rh sensitization; Rh immunization: The process of being sensitized to the Rh factor. Experimentally, it has been found (Wiener) that the most effective way to immunize Rh-negative subjects is to inject small doses, e.g., 2 cc. of Rh-positive blood at 4-month intervals. The first injection acts as a primer, and after the second injection more than 40 per cent of the subjects become immunized. If the injections are continued, more than 75 per cent of Rh-negative persons can be immunized, while a small minority of individuals appear to be relatively incapable of responding to the injections. Under clinical conditions, therefore, two widely spaced transfusions of Rh-positive blood are more likely to lead to Rh sensitization than multiple large transfusions in a short space of time. Moreover, it has been found that fetal blood enters the maternal circulation during the course of approximately one out of three normal pregnancies and one out of three deliveries. This helps to explain why erythroblastosis fetalis occurs generally in only one out of twenty of the second-born infants of Rh-negative mothers. Once a person has been sensitized to the Rh factor, he remains so for the remainder of his life, though the antibody titer tends to fall gradually with the passage of time.

Preparation of Rh-Hr typing serum: The deliberate immunization of volunteer male donors is an innocuous procedure which has been successfully applied for the preparation of diagnostic conglutinating serum. However, the method has not proved practicable for the production of agglutinating anti-Rh_0 or of Rh-Hr antisera of specificities other than anti-Rh_0. These latter reagents, therefore, become available only when a relatively rare patient becomes sensitized by transfusion or pregnancy. Before such sera can be used, they must be absorbed to remove any alpha or beta isoagglutinins that they may contain, using group A and group B red cells of the appropriate Rh-Hr type.

Absorption of antisera: A method of removing antibodies from a polyvalent serum in order to render it monovalent and type specific. The most common practical application of the technic is for the preparation of blood typing sera, and to resolve clinical problems of multiple isosensitization. For purifying anti-Rh_0 serum from a group O person, for example, pooled, washed and packed A_1 rh and B rh cells are added to the serum and the mixture is allowed to stand for about an hour. The mixture is then centrifuged, the serum recovered, and the process repeated as many times as necessary to render the serum specific. The method is also useful to determine whether a serum reacting with a variety of bloods contains a mixture of antibodies separable by absorption or a single antibody detecting a common blood factor. For example, some antisera which react on blood having either factor Rh_0 or rh′ are truly polyvalent, and are therefore designated anti-Rh_0′. Other such sera exist, however, without separable antibodies and are designated anti-rh^G, since they detect a blood factor rh^G shared by blood having either factor Rh_0 or rh′. It is clear that designations such as anti-**A**+**B**+**C**, etc. are misleading, if not incorrect, unless the sera actually contain antibodies anti-**A**, anti-**B**, etc., separable by absorption.

Non-specific absorption: A term sometimes applied to "explain" the difficulty of purifying certain antisera by absorption. For example, in the preparation of anti-A_1 serum by absorption of serum from group B individuals with A_2 cells, and in the preparation of anti-**N** serum by absorption with type M cells, use of an excess of cells can destroy the reactivity of the reagent completely, due to "non-specific over-absorption." The explanation may be that the difference between A_1 and A_2 and between M and N is not as sharp as between Rh-negative and Rh-positive blood—that is, A_2 cells have A_1-like blood factors, and type M cells have **N**-like blood factors.

Elution: The reverse of absorption. The method was first applied by Landsteiner and Miller for "purification" of auto-antibodies and alpha and beta isoagglutinins, which were absorbed onto red cells at refrigerator temperature and then eluted into saline solutions at body temperature or higher (56 C.). A similar method has been applied for purifying Rh-Hr antibodies but because of the high temperatures required for elution, the eluate often contains hemoglobin and is unpleasant to work with. Therefore, many workers use the following method recommended by W. Weiner:

After sensitization, the cells are washed four to six times with iced saline solution. The cells are then frozen and thawed until lysed, and then about five volumes of 50 per cent cold (−20 C.) ethyl alcohol are added. The mixture is kept at −20 C. for at least 30 minutes, centrifuged and the supernatant discarded. To the sediment, saline or serum or bovine albumin solution is added, and the mixture kept at body temperature for at least 30 minutes. The supernate recovered by centrifugation should contain the eluted antibody.

Anamnestic reaction: The exaggerated response to the injection of an antigen which occurs in a previously immunized subject. For example, in a sensitized Rh-negative person whose antibody titer has fallen after the passage of many years, an injection of a small amount of Rh-positive blood will stimulate a pronounced and sustained rise in antibody titer. That is why even though the Rh antibody titer may be low or zero at the beginning of a pregnancy, the prognosis for the Rh-positive baby remains uncertain—leakage of a small amount of Rh-positive blood into the maternal circulation from the fetus *in utero*, such as may occur in one out of three pregnancies, may stimulate a marked rise in titer in a previously primed Rh-negative pregnant woman. Reports that pregnancies, even with Rh-negative babies, can cause a "non-specific" anamnestic rise in titer are erroneous and appear to be based on inaccurate titrations or too literal interpretation of the results of titrations which have a large experimental error. When more careful titrations are done, non-specific anamnestic reactions do not occur. To accept reports of such reactions at face value is tantamount to believing that specific Rh antisera can be produced by injecting Rh-negative subjects with Rh-negative blood.

A practical application of this phenomenon is in the production of Rh-Hr and other antisera. When individuals who have antibodies of an unusual specificity, but too weak for the preparation of useful diagnostic reagents, are given an injection of a small amount of incompatible blood, this may act as a booster and produce a valuable antiserum.

Tests for Rh sensitization: Tests on the serum of Rh-negative individuals to determine the presence or absence of Rh antibodies. Such tests should be carried out on all pregnant Rh-negative women, except those with Rh-negative husbands, in order to anticipate the possible occurrence of erythroblastosis fetalis in the baby. In primiparas, Rh sensitization is not apt to occur unless the expectant mother has been primed by a transfusion or an intramuscular injection of Rh-positive blood, though erythroblastosis sometimes occurs in primiparas in the absence of such a history. In multiparas, the tests for Rh antibodies should be carried out at stated intervals throughout the pregnancy, and should be so designed as to detect univalent as well as bivalent antibodies. Rh-positive persons can also be sensitized; e.g., type Rh_1Rh_1 individuals can become sensitized to the **rh″** factor or the **hr′** factor or both. Such cases are relatively rare, however.

Rh agglutination test: A test for bivalent Rh antibodies (*cf.* fig. 4). This may be carried out as follows: Three 2 per cent saline suspensions are prepared of fresh blood from group O individuals of types Rh_1, Rh_2, and rh. One drop of the type Rh_1 cell suspension is placed in a small tube, a drop of Rh_2 cells in a second tube, and a drop of type rh cells in a third tube; to each tube a drop of the patient's serum is added. The mixtures are incubated at body temperature for 1 hour and the reactions read by inspecting the pattern of the sediment (Landsteiner and Wiener), or, after gentle shaking, the mixture is examined for the presence or absence of clumping. The reactions can generally be accentuated by light centrifugation (500 rpm for 1 minute). Clumping of the type Rh_1 and type Rh_2 cells, but not of the type rh cells, indicates the presence of Rh sensitization.

Rh blocking test (***Wiener***): A test to detect Rh antibodies of the univalent variety (*cf.* fig. 4). This test is carried out in two stages, the first being the same as the agglutination test. If the test for Rh_0 agglutinins is negative, then a drop of anti-Rh_0 agglutinating serum of moderate titer (10 to 20 units) is added to the mixture of patient's serum and Rh-positive cells. The mixtures are then incubated for an additional 1 to 2 hours at body temperature, and failure of clumping to occur indicates the presence of Rh_0 blocking antibodies in the patient's serum. This is the least sensitive test for univalent antibodies, for unless the antibodies are of relatively high titer and avidity, they will not coat enough Rh loci on the test cells for blocking to result. For this reason, when the blocking test for Rh antibodies is positive, this indicates a high titer of univalent antibodies, and in the case of an Rh-negative mother who is bearing an Rh-positive fetus, the prognosis for the infant is generally grave, and stillbirths are not uncommon.

Rh conglutination test (Wiener): An important test to detect Rh antibodies of the univalent type (*cf.* fig. 5). This test can be carried out in two stages or in one stage. In the two-stage method, the first stage is the agglutination test. If the agglutination test is negative, the tubes are centrifuged and the supernatant removed as completely as possible with a fine capillary pipette. Then one or two large drops of undiluted pooled oxalated plasma, or, better, a mixture of 3 or 4 parts plasma and 1 part of 30 per cent bovine albumin (or 25 per cent human albumin) are added and the cells resuspended. After a second period of incubation, the tubes are shaken and the reactions read. In the one-stage method, the testing cells are suspended in 20 per cent bovine albumin instead of saline solution. One drop of the patient's serum is mixed with a drop of albumin-suspended test cells; the mixtures are incubated at body temperature and the reactions then read. The conglutination test is considerably more sensitive than the blocking test for the detection of univalent Rh antibodies.

Anti-globulin test for Rh antibodies; indirect Coombs' test: A sensitive two-stage test for univalent Rh antibodies, based on the principle that such antibodies are modified gamma globulins (*cf.* fig. 6). For the test a special reagent, anti-human globulin serum, is needed. Anti-human globulin serum is prepared by immunizing rabbits or other animals with human serum of group O, or with purified human gamma globulin. Heteroagglutinins for human red cells are removed from serum of satisfactory titer by absorbing it with packed pooled human red cells freed of human plasma by washing seven or more times with large volumes of saline solution. The anti-globulin test for Rh antibodies is carried out in two stages. In the first stage, a drop of the patient's serum is mixed with a drop of saline suspension of red cells, and the mixture is incubated at body temperature. The sensitized cells are then washed three or four times

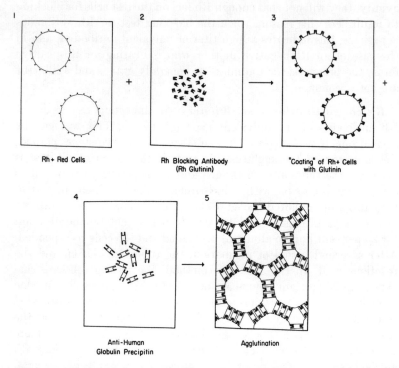

FIG. 6.—Diagrammatic visualization of the antiglobulin test. (Wiener, A. S.: This Month in American Medicine, January 1947).

with an excess of saline solution in order to remove all traces of human globulin which could inhibit the anti-globulin serum. To the washed red cell sediment a drop of anti-globulin serum is added, and the mixture centrifuged at 500 rpm for 1 minute, the tube gently shaken and the reaction read. Clumping of Rh-positive cells, but not of Rh-negative cells, indicates that the patient is sensitized to the Rh factor.

Anti-human globulin serum; Coombs' serum: The reagent used in the anti-globulin or Coombs' test. This is generally prepared by immunizing rabbits, although satisfactory reagents have also been obtained by immunizing larger animals, notably goats. Two varieties have been described, anti-gamma globulin and anti-non-gamma globulin serum. The former is more readily prepared and is the kind used in Rh-Hr tests. The anti-non-gamma globulin sera appear to be directed against some thermolabile component of the serum, complement-like in nature, and are used for tests with antibodies of the Kidd blood group system, anti-Lewis antibodies, and certain cold-reacting antibodies such as anti-**H**.

Proteolytic enzyme test for Rh antibodies (*Morton and Pickles*): A most sensitive test for univalent antibodies, based on the principle that after treatment with proteolytic enzymes such as trypsin, papain, ficin, and bromelin, saline suspensions of Rh-positive cells undergo strong specific clumping when mixed with sera containing univalent Rh antibodies. In the authors' hands, best results have been obtained with the enzymes ficin and papain. In order to enzyme-treat cells, they are first washed with saline solution to remove plasma which contains enzyme inhibitor; then nine parts of packed cells are mixed with one part of a 1 per cent solution of ficin (or papain) and incubated at body temperature for 60 to 90 minutes. The action of the enzyme is stopped by washing with saline solution, and a suspension of the enzyme-treated cells in saline solution is prepared. The test for Rh antibodies is carried out in the same way as the agglutination test, using a suspension of enzyme-treated cells instead of unmodified cells.

The mechanism of this test is not entirely clear (*cf.* fig. 7). Proteolytic enzymes do not appear to affect the Rh loci, but to act on the anti-sphering substance (crystalbumin) on the red cells' surface. As a result, the net negative surface charge is reduced, as shown by the reduced mobility of the cells in an electrophoretic field (Ponder), and the cells become more agglutinable. The proteolytic enzymes do not damage the A-B-O agglutinogens, but they do affect the M-N agglutinogens, so that the test cannot be used to detect **M** and **N** antibodies.

The agglutination, conglutination, anti-globulin and enzyme-treated cells technic can be used for detecting any of the known Rh-Hr antibodies. The anti-globulin method is the only satisfactory technic for detecting univalent **F** (Duffy) antibodies; this may be due to the apparently smaller number of antigenic loci for this blood group system on the discoplasm. The anti-globulin

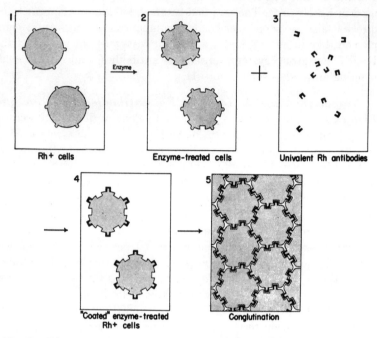

FIG. 7.—Diagrammatic visualization of the reaction of univalent Rh antibodies with enzyme-treated Rh-positive cells. (Wiener, A. S., and Katz, L. J.: Immunol. *66:* 51, 1951.)

test is the most satisfactory for detecting the causes of intragroup incompatibilities when analyzing blood transfusion problems. For detecting **K** (Kell) antibodies, either the conglutination or the anti-globulin test may be used.

Titration: Determining the quantity of antibody in a serum. Unlike chemical titrations, serological titrations have a large intrinsic error, so that variations as great as 100 or even 200 per cent are not unusual, even in the hands of experts. Satisfactory results can, however, be obtained by taking all readings blind, and averaging the results of several titrations. In the usual technic, the test cells are mixed with progressively doubled dilutions of the serum in a series of small tubes, and the highest dilution giving a distinct positive reaction is determined.

Blind test: A method in which one worker sets up the test and a second independent worker reads the reactions without knowing the identity of the mixtures. The method is essential to insure objectivity in determining the end points of titrations, and in carrying out tests with antisera of low titer and avidity, such as anti-**H**, anti-**Le**, anti-**F**, and anti-**J** (Kidd). Failure to use the blind technic has led to erroneous reports which could not be confirmed by other workers, such as the claims for the discovery of anti-**Hr**$_0$.

Titer of serum: The concentration of a specific antibody in an antiserum; the potency of an antiserum. This is usually expressed in units, which are calculated by taking the reciprocal of the highest dilution of serum giving a distinct (1 plus) reaction under the conditions of the test. When giving the titer of a serum, the technic of titration must be stated, since the sensitivities of the different methods are not the same. For example, an average univalent anti-**Rh**$_0$ serum with a titer of 1 unit by the blocking method may have a titer of about 20 units by the albumin-plasma conglutination method, 50 units by the anti-globulin method, and 100 units or higher for ficinated red cells. The literature contains many reports of fantastically high titers running into the tens of millions units, caused by carrying over. (In our own hands, among tens of thousands of antibody titrations, no antibody titer exceeding 200,000 units has ever been encountered.) Carrying over can be avoided by using a fresh pipette for each dilution, or rinsing thoroughly with a fresh tube of diluent solution between dilutions. Moreover, every extraordinarily high titer should be confirmed by accurately preparing a 1:10 or 1:100 dilution of the serum and then titrating this diluted serum.

Rh$_0$ blocking serum: An **Rh**$_0$ antiserum containing univalent antibodies of sufficiently high titer and avidity to give clear-cut blocking reactions. Such sera are useful for blocking anti-**Rh**$_0'$ agglutinating serums to prepare anti-**rh'** reagents, and for blocking anti-**Rh**$_0''$ agglutinating serums in order to prepare anti-**rh''** reagents. Since Rh-positive cells that are blocked by **Rh**$_0$ univalent antibodies can still react with anti-**rh'** and anti-**rh''** sera, it appears that the blood factor **Rh**$_0$ is associated with an aspect of the agglutinogen molecule separate from factors **rh'** and **rh''**, and that the active patch for the **Rh**$_0$ blocking antibody molecule is smaller than the complete

Rh-Hr agglutinogen molecule. Moreover, because of their ability to pass across the intact placental barrier, **Rh$_0$** blocking antibodies are thought to be smaller than the **Rh$_0$** agglutinating antibodies, which are held back by the intact placenta.

CHAPTER III

Immunogenetics of the Rh-Hr Blood Types

Phenotypes: The characteristics of individuals as determined by direct observation, measurement, chemical or serological testing, etc. Thus, the characteristics, blue eyes, tall, short, hemophiliac, group O, type MN, Rh positive, type Rh_1Rh_2, etc., are all phenotypes. The phenotypes may be partially or wholly genetically determined, or may be entirely determined by the environment; e.g., the color of the hair is usually genetically determined, but it changes with age, and can be completely changed by dyeing. An environmentally determined characteristic which resembles one that is genetically determined has been termed a phenocopy.

Genotypes: The constitutional make-up of an individual as determined by heredity. The genotype is transmitted through the germ cells by means of their chromosomes, though there is evidence also, in exceptional cases, of cytoplasmic inheritance. According to the gene theory, each of the 23 pairs of chromosomes contains numerous genes, the units of heredity, arranged in linear order. With only the exception of the genes on the sex chromosomes in the male, every individual has a pair of every kind of gene in his somatic cells (as would be expected from the fact that chromosomes occur in pairs), one derived from the maternal parent, the other from the paternal parent. The make-up of the individual in terms of his genes is known as his genotype.

Rh_0 phenotypes: The two phenotypes, Rh positive and Rh negative, which can be distinguished with the aid of anti-Rh_0 serum. This is the most important classification of individuals as far as the Rh factor is concerned, since **Rh_0** is the most antigenic of the Rh-Hr blood factors, and therefore the most common source of clinical complications.

29

Rh_0 genotypes: The three genotypes, *Rh Rh*, *Rh rh* and *rh rh* are based on the theory that the **Rh_0** factor is inherited as a simple mendelian dominant by means of a pair of allelic genes, *Rh* and *rh*. Thus, Rh-negative individuals are always homozygous (genotype *rh rh*), and if they intermarry, produce only Rh-negative children. Rh-positive individuals, on the other hand, may be homozygous (genotype *Rh Rh*) or heterozygous (genotype *Rh rh*).

Homozygous: Of a genotype consisting of two identical genes. If an Rh-negative expectant mother has a homozygous Rh-positive husband, all of their children will be Rh positive.

Heterozygous: Of a genotype consisting of two different genes. If an Rh-negative expectant mother has a heterozygous Rh-positive husband, half of their children will be Rh positive, and half will be Rh negative.

Hypothetic anti-Hr_0 serum: A hypothetic serum giving reactions with the product of gene *rh*, and therefore reciprocally related to **Rh_0**. If anti-**Hr_0** were available, three phenotypes could be distinguished, corresponding to the three theoretically possible genotypes, as follows:

Phenotypes	Reactions with		Genotypes
	Anti-Rh_0	Anti-Hr_0	
Rh positive			
Rh_0..............................	+	−	*Rh Rh*
Rh_0Hr_0.........................	+	+	*Rh rh*
Rh negative: Hr_0..................	−	+	*rh rh*

Anti-**Hr_0** serum has never been found, but useful genetic information can be obtained with the aid of anti-**hr'** and anti-**hr''** sera (*cf.* page 37).

Rh-rh gene frequencies: The incidence of the genes *Rh* and *rh* in the general population can be calculated from the distribution of the **Rh_0** factor. Since Rh-negative individuals are always homozygous, genotype *rh rh*, $rh = \sqrt{\text{Rh neg.}}$, and $Rh = 1 - rh$. For example, since approximately 15 per cent of Caucasians are Rh negative, $rh = \sqrt{0.15}$ = approximately 40 per cent, and Rh = 60 per cent.

Factors Rh^A, Rh^B, Rh^C, Rh^D, etc.: Blood factors almost regularly associated with the blood factor Rh_0 of Rh-positive blood. The existence of these factors was discovered when Rh-positive patients were encountered who had become isosensitized, and had antibodies in their serum almost indistinguishable from anti-Rh_0 in specificity. Clearly, the antibodies in question were not the common anti-Rh_0, however, since the sera failed to react with the patient's own red cells, and also did not react with certain other rare Rh-positive bloods. Furthermore, comparison of sera from different cases showed that not all gave parallel reactions, indicating that they were detecting different blood factors. This makes necessary the use of a distinctive symbol for each such newly found blood factor. Theoretically, the number of such factors is unlimited, and at least four have been shown to exist. When Rh-positive blood is shown to lack one or more of the associated factors, this is indicated by the use of an appropriate superscript small letter, e.g., an individual of type Rh^{cd} is Rh positive but lacks factors Rh^C and Rh^D. Such a person, if transfused with ordinary compatible Rh-positive blood, could become sensitized to factor Rh^C or factor Rh^D or both. It must be emphasized that such individuals are rare, and in routine Rh_0 testing give the usual positive reactions. Their existence, therefore, is only detected when they become isosensitized either by transfusion or pregnancy. Bloods of type Rh^{ab}, Rh^d, etc., must be distinguished from the more common Rh_0-variant blood (*cf.* page 43).

The eight Rh phenotypes: The eight types of blood that can be distinguished with the aid of sera anti-Rh_0, anti-rh′ and anti-rh″. These are set forth in table 3.

Separate pairs of genes vs. multiple alleles: When blood factors Rh_0 and rh′ were discovered in 1941, the question arose whether these were inherited by separate pairs of genes, or whether the factors were attributes of complex agglutinogens inherited by a series of multiple allelic genes. If there were a separate pair of allelic genes for factor rh′ and a separate gene pair for factor Rh_0, these two pairs of genes could either be independent (i.e., in different pairs of chromosomes), or linked (in the same chromosome). By independent assortment or crossing over, equilibrium must have been reached after many thousands of generations. If separate gene pairs were

involved, the following relationship among the four possible phenotypes would therefore have to hold:*

$$(\mathbf{Rh}_0 + \mathbf{rh'}+) \times (\mathbf{Rh}_0 - \mathbf{rh'}-) = (\mathbf{Rh}_0 + \mathbf{rh'}-) \times (\mathbf{Rh}_0 - \mathbf{rh'}+)$$

or, expressed in terms of the frequencies of the eight Rh phenotypes:

$$(Rh_1 + Rh_Z) \times (rh + rh'') = (Rh_0 + Rh_2) \times (rh' + rh_y).$$

Since this relationship does not hold in any population, Wiener was
led, as early as 1942, to discard the concept of separate gene pairs and
to adopt the theory of multiple alleles.

Thus, the theory of linked genes to account for the inheritance of
the Rh types, whether by gene couplets, or by triply or quadruply
linked genes (Fisher and Race) is merely an elaboration of a theory
previously disproved and discarded by Wiener.

Theory of multiple alleles (Wiener): To account for the Rh
types, rh, rh', rh'', and Rh_0, four corresponding allelic genes, r, r', r'',
and R^0 are required. Moreover, in certain families where one parent
is of type rh and the other is type Rh_1, the children are almost
invariably either type Rh_1 or type rh, indicating that in such cases
the factors $\mathbf{Rh}_0$ and $\mathbf{rh'}$ are attributes of one and the same agglutinogen. It is necessary therefore to postulate a unit agglutinogen Rh_1
(having both factors $\mathbf{Rh}_0$ and $\mathbf{rh'}$) inherited by a corresponding allelic
gene R^1. Similarly, it is necessary to postulate a unit agglutinogen
Rh_2 (with the blood factors $\mathbf{Rh}_0$ and $\mathbf{rh''}$) and a corresponding allelic
gene R^2. The resulting theory of six allelic genes, r, r', r'', R^0, R^1, and
R^2, leads to 21 possible genotypes, corresponding to the eight phenotypes, as shown in table 6. Actually, it is necessary to postulate a
minimum of eight allelic genes, but the six-gene theory is a useful
approximation for many purposes.

Allelic genes; allelomorphic genes: Alternative genes situated
at corresponding loci in a pair of chromosomes. Genes which influence
different specific characteristics, such as the A-B-O groups, the
M-N-S types, the Rh-Hr types, eye color, etc., are located at different
specific loci. All the alternative genes that can occur at a given locus
are known as allelic genes. Since the locus for the allelic genes of the
A-B-O groups is on a different pair of chromosomes from the allelic
genes of the M-N-S types, while the allelic genes of the Rh-Hr

---

* In the formula, $(\mathbf{Rh}_0 + \mathbf{rh'}+)$ represents the frequency of bloods possessing
both blood factors $\mathbf{Rh}_0$ and $\mathbf{rh'}$; $(\mathbf{Rh}_0 + \mathbf{rh'}-)$ represents blood with factor $\mathbf{Rh}_0$
but lacking $\mathbf{rh'}$; etc.

TABLE 6.—*The Six-Allele Theory of Inheritance of the Rh Types*

Phenotype*	Corresponding Genotypes
rh	rr
rh′	$r'r'$ and $r'r$
rh″	$r''r''$ and $r''r$
rh$_y$	$r'r''$
Rh$_0$	R^0R^0 and R^0r
Rh$_1$	R^1R^1, R^1r', R^1r, R^1R^0, and R^0r'
Rh$_2$	R^2R^2, R^2r'', R^2r, R^2R^0, and R^0r''
Rh$_z$	R^1R^2, R^1r'', and R^2r'

* Phenotype rh$_y$ was formerly designated rh′rh″, while phenotype Rh$_z$ was formerly designated phenotype Rh$_1$Rh$_2$.

system are on a third pair of chromosomes, these three blood group systems are inherited independently of one another. This is supported by family studies and the observation that the distribution of the Rh types is the same among individuals of any A-B-O group (e.g., among group O individuals), or among individuals of any M-N-S type (e.g., type N.S), as in the general population. The distribution of the Rh types is also the same in the two sexes, indicating that the Rh locus is not on the sex chromosomes, a conclusion that has been confirmed by family studies.

Linked genes: When nonallelic genes for two distinct characteristics are on the same pair of chromosomes, they are said to be linked; if they are on different chromosomes, they are said to be independent.

Rh gene frequencies: From the distribution of the eight Rh types in the general population, the frequencies of the six principal Rh genes can be calculated (Wiener) with the aid of the following formulae:

$$r = \sqrt{\text{rh}} \tag{1}$$

$$r' = \sqrt{\text{rh}'+\text{rh}} - \sqrt{\text{rh}} \tag{2}$$

$$r'' = \sqrt{\text{rh}''+\text{rh}} - \sqrt{\text{rh}} \tag{3}$$

$$R^0 = \sqrt{\text{Rh}_0+\text{rh}} - \sqrt{\text{rh}} \tag{4}$$

$$R^1 = \sqrt{\text{Rh}_1+\text{rh}'+\text{Rh}_0+\text{rh}} - \sqrt{\text{rh}'+\text{rh}} - \sqrt{\text{Rh}_0+\text{rh}} + \sqrt{\text{rh}} \tag{5}$$

$$R^2 = \sqrt{\text{Rh}_2+\text{rh}''+\text{Rh}_0+\text{rh}} - \sqrt{\text{rh}''+\text{rh}} - \sqrt{\text{Rh}_0+\text{rh}} + \sqrt{\text{rh}} \tag{6}$$

The sum of the gene frequencies as calculated by these formulae closely approximates 100 per cent, and this an important part of the evidence supporting the theory of multiple alleles. Actually, the sum of the gene frequencies falls short of 100 per cent, because of the existence of the additional allelic genes r^y and R^z. The genes r^y and R^z are so rare, however, that they have no noticeable effect on such calculations (*cf.* table 8).

Family studies on the eight Rh types: These provide additional evidence of the correctness of the multiple allele theory, as shown by Wiener's studies on 1,346 families with 2,221 children (table 7). Aside from two apparent exceptions to the theory which are caused by illegitimacy, there are a few inconsistencies with the six-gene theory in the matings rh $\times$ Rh$_z$ and rh $\times$ rh$_y$. According to the six-gene theory, a parent of type Rh$_z$ (genotypes R^1R^2, R^1r'', or R^2r') cannot have a type rh child (genotype rr); nor can a type rh parent have a type Rh$_z$ child; similarly, the parent-child combination rh$_y$ $\rightleftarrows$ rh should not occur. Such exceptions to the six-gene theory are due to the existence of the two additional rare genes R^z and r^y (*cf.* table 8).

The rare genes r^y and R^Z: Two additional rare allelic Rh genes, which account for contradictions to the six-gene theory. The gene R^Z has a frequency of only 1/10 per cent (*cf.* table 8), and gives rise to a corresponding agglutinogen Rh$_z$ with all three Rh factors, **Rh$_0$**, **rh'**, and **rh''**; gene r^y is even rarer (1/100 per cent) and gives rise to an agglutinogen rh$_y$ with the factors **rh'** and **rh''**, but lacking factor **Rh$_0$**. Families illustrating the transmission of the rare genes R^Z and r^y are given in table 9.

Family studies: multiple alleles vs. separate gene pairs: Family studies offer another opportunity to test the relative merits of the theory of multiple alleles as opposed to separate gene pairs. In families in which one parent belongs to type rh, according to the theory of multiple alleles no more than two different Rh types can occur among children in any one family. According to the theory of triple gene pairs, on the other hand, by crossing over, as many as eight different Rh phenotypes could occur in the same family. Significantly, to date, no more than two Rh types have occurred in such matings. If one argues that linkage is so tight that crossing over

TABLE 7.—*Author's Studies on the Heredity of the Eight Rh Types*
(1943–1953)

Mating	No. of Families	Number of Children of Type								Total
		rh	rh'	rh''	rhy	Rho	Rh1	Rh2	Rhz	
rh × rh	32	53	0	0	0	0	0	0	0	53
rh × rh'	3	1	2	0	0	0	0	(1)	0	4
rh × rh''	2	2	0	5	0	0	0	0	0	7
rh × rhy	1	1	0	0	1	0	0	0	0	2
rh × Rho	31	15	0	0	0	33	0	0	0	48
rh × Rh1	599	182	5	0	0	40	731	(1)	0	959
rh × Rh2	126	72	0	0	0	4	0	144	0	220
rh × Rhz	152	3	1	0	0	0	112	120	7	243
rh' × Rho	3	0	2	0	0	1	2	0	0	5
rh' × Rh1	31	7	7	0	0	5	30	0	0	49
rh' × Rh2	8	2	5	0	0	0	0	3	3	13
rh' × Rhz	10	0	0	0	0	0	6	4	7	17
rh'' × Rh1	14	3	0	1	0	0	8	0	11	23
rh'' × Rh2	3	0	0	2	0	0	0	3	0	5
rh'' × Rhz	4	0	0	0	0	0	2	0	2	4
rhy × Rho	1	0	0	3	0	0	0	0	0	3
rhy × Rh1	2	0	0	0	0	0	1	0	2	3
rhy × Rh2	1	0	0	0	0	0	0	1	1	2
Rho × Rho	1	0	0	0	0	1	0	0	0	1
Rho × Rh1	19	6	1	0	0	4	16	0	0	27
Rho × Rh2	4	1	0	0	0	4	0	2	0	7
Rho × Rhz	3	0	0	0	0	0	2	1	0	3
Rh1 × Rh1	125	12	1	0	0	6	188	0	0	207
Rh1 × Rh2	57	12	4	0	0	5	35	13	29	98
Rh1 × Rhz	71	0	1	0	0	0	74	17	53	145
Rh2 × Rh2	10	3	0	0	0	0	0	13	0	16
Rh2 × Rhz	18	0	0	0	0	0	8	17	12	37
Rhz × Rhz	14	0	0	0	0	0	6	4	8	18
ℜh1 × Rhz	1	0	0	0	0	0	2	0	0	2
Totals	1346	375	29	11	1	103	1223	344	135	2221

The numbers in parentheses represent contradictions to the genetic theory, apparently due to illegitimacy.

These data include material compiled during the years 1943 to 1953. More recently it has been found that about 40 per cent of blood specimens previously classified as type rh' actually belong to type ℜh₁, since they contain a weakly reacting **Rh₀** factor (ℜh₀). The technic has recently been changed so as to determine factor ℜh₀ (see last line of table), but it must be borne in mind that many of the individuals in this table classified as type rh' may actually be type ℜh₁.

The excess of families with Rh-negative parents is explained by the fact that this material was largely compiled from families confronted with the problem of Rh sensitization.

TABLE 8.—*The Rh Series of Allelic Genes*

Genes	Frequencies among N.Y.C. Caucasoids (per cent)	Corresponding Agglutinogens	Reactions with Rh Antisera*			Reactions with Hr Antisera		
			Anti-Rh_0	Anti-rh'	Anti-rh''	Anti-hr'	Anti-hr''	Anti-hr
r	38.0	rh	−	−	−	+	+	+
r'	1.4	rh'	−	+	−	−	+	−
r''	0.5	rh''	−	−	+	+	−	−
r^y	.01	rh_y	−	+	+	−	−	−
R^0	3.2	Rh_0	+	−	−	+	+	+
R^1	40.4	Rh_1	+	+	−	−	+	−
R^2	16.4	Rh_2	+	−	+	+	−	−
R^Z	0.1	Rh_z	+	+	+	−	−	−

* The individual's phenotype is the result of the action of a pair of genes; e.g., genotype R^1R^2, genotype R^1r, etc. The effect of a single gene can be inferred however from the study of homozygous individuals, e.g., rr, R^1R^1, R^2R^2, etc. In the case of the rare genes r', r'', R^Z and r^y, where homozygous individuals are not readily available, the effect of the individual gene is determined by deduction.

is never observed, then actually the supposed triply linked genes behave as a unit, as in the theory of multiple alleles.

Subtyping for rh^w factor (Callender and Race): With the aid of anti-**rh^w** serum a further subdivision of the eight Rh types is

TABLE 9.—*Families Illustrating the Transmission of the Rare Genes R^Z and r^y*

Mating	Children				
	1	2	3	4	5
1. $Rh_z \times rh$	rh	Rh_z			
$R^Zr \times rr$	rr	R^Zr			
2. $rh_y \times rh$	rh	rh_y			
$r^yr \times rr$	rr	r^yr			
3. $Rh_z \times rh$	rh	rh	Rh_z	rh	Rh_z
$R^Zr \times rr$	rr	rr	R^zr	rr	R^zr

possible. The **rh**^{w} (or **rh**^{w1}) factor occurs in approximately 5 per cent of Caucasoids, and always in association with factor **rh**$'$. Thus, the type Rh$_1$ is subdivided into Rh$^w_1$ and Rh$_1$ proper, while type Rh$_1$Rh$_2$ (or Rh$_z$) is subdivided into Rh$^w_1$Rh$_2$ (or Rh^w_z) and Rh$_1$Rh$_2$ (or Rh$_z$) proper. Therefore, there are two main forms of Rh$_1$ agglutinogen, namely, Rh$^w_1$ and Rh$_1$ proper, inherited by corresponding allelic genes R^{1w} and R^1. A similar subdivision of type rh$'$ and type rh$'$rh$''$ (rh$_y$) also exists, but only a small number of persons of the rare type rh$'^w$ have been encountered to date. The practical importance of the **rh**^{w} factor is to explain rare puzzling examples of erythroblastosis fetalis where both mother and baby are of type Rh$_1$, namely, by showing the baby to be of subtype Rh$^w_1$ and the mother sensitized to the **rh**^{w} factor. Similarly, **rh**^{w} sensitization accounts for certain rare intragroup hemolytic transfusion reactions. Anti-**rh**^{w} sera are generally obtained from the rare sensitized patients, but have also been produced by deliberate immunization of volunteer donors.

Anti-Hr sera: Antisera specific for the Hr factors. Such antisera are much rarer than Rh antisera, because in general the Hr factors are considerably less antigenic than the Rh factors; in fact, attempts to produce anti-Hr sera by immunizing volunteers has met with little or no success. Two principal anti-Hr sera are available, namely, anti-**hr**$'$ and anti-**hr**$''$, which are so named because of their reciprocal relationship to anti-**rh**$'$ and anti-**rh**$''$, respectively. The reactions of the Hr sera are shown in simplified form in table 10 (eight-gene theory), and in greater detail in table 11 (ten-gene theory). As can be seen, the main practical value of anti-**hr**$'$ serum is for subdividing type Rh$_1$ individuals into the two types Rh$_1$Rh$_1$ and Rh$_1$rh, while in the same way anti-**hr**$''$ serum subdivides Rh$_2$ type into types Rh$_2$Rh$_2$ and Rh$_2$rh. In this way a *presumptive* diagnosis of homozygosity and heterozygosity is possible when typing husbands of Rh-negative expectant mothers, a matter of considerable practical importance in anticipating the possible occurrence of erythroblastosis in the unborn child. Anti-**hr**$''$ sera are much rarer than anti-**hr**$'$ sera, since **hr**$''$ is less antigenic. A serum with the specificity anti-**Hr**$_0$ would be most valuable for determining zygosity (with respect to factor **Rh**$_0$) but unfortunately does not exist (*cf.* page 30); instead, a serum of a different specificity, anti-**hr**, has been found (*cf.* tables 8 and 11).

Rh-Hr types; Rh-Hr phenotypes: Types of human blood demonstrable by the combined use of Rh and Hr antisera. The

Table 10.—*Wiener's Nomenclature of the 18 Rh-Hr Blood Types and 36 Genotypes*

| Eight Rh Phenotypes | Reactions with Serum | | Designation | |
	Anti-hr'	Anti-hr''	Phenotypes	Corresponding genotypes
rh	+	+	rh	rr
rh'	+	+	rh'rh	$r'r$
	−	+	rh'rh'	$r'r'$
rh''	+	+	rh''rh	$r''r$
	+	−	rh''rh''	$r''r''$
rh$_y$ (or rh'rh'')	+	+	rh$_y$rh	$r'r''$ and $r^y r$
	−	+	rh$_y$rh'	$r^y r'$
	+	−	rh$_y$rh''	$r^y r''$
	−	−	rh$_y$rh$_y$	$r^y r^y$
Rh$_0$	+	+	Rh$_0$	$R^0 R^0$ and $R^0 r$
Rh$_1$	+	+	Rh$_1$rh	$R^1 r$, $R^1 R^0$ and $R^0 r'$
	−	+	Rh$_1$Rh$_1$	$R^1 R^1$ and $R^1 r'$
Rh$_2$	+	+	Rh$_2$rh	$R^2 r$, $R^2 R^0$, and $R^0 r''$
	+	−	Rh$_2$Rh$_2$	$R^2 R^2$ and $R^2 r''$
Rh$_z$ (or Rh$_1$Rh$_2$)	+	+	Rh$_z$Rh$_0$	$R^1 R^2$, $R^1 r''$, $R^2 r'$, $R^z r$, $R^z R^0$ and $R^0 r^y$
	−	+	Rh$_z$Rh$_1$	$R^z R^1$, $R^z r'$, and $R^1 r^y$
	+	−	Rh$_z$Rh$_2$	$R^z R^2$, $R^z r''$, and $R^2 r^y$
	−	−	Rh$_z$Rh$_z$	$R^z R^z$ and $R^z r^y$

number of phenotypes which can be differentiated of necessity depends on the number of different antisera used in the tests, and the evolution of knowledge as more antisera became available is summarized in table 11. With anti-**hr** serum in short supply, the examination is generally confined to tests for the three "standard" Rh factors and to tests for **hr'** and **hr''**, under which circumstances 18 phenotypes can be distinguished (*cf.* table 10). (If tests are carried out for the **rh**^{w} factor also, the number of recognizable phenotypes will be increased, as is shown in table 11.) It should be emphasized that many of the phenotypes are quite rare, especially those involving the agglutinogens rh′, rh″, rh_y and Rh_z. In order that the symbols for the phenotypes indicate what tests have actually been carried out, the principle is employed that the first of the two symbols in the name shall represent the reactions of the Rh antisera, while the second symbol in the phenotype name represents the reactions with Hr antisera. For example, Rh_2rh represents positive reactions with Rh antisera anti-**Rh**₀ and anti-**rh″**, but not with anti-**rh′** (Rh_2 = Rh_0 + rh″), and with both Hr antisera anti-**hr′** and anti-**hr″** (rh = **hr′** and hr″).

The phenotype corresponding to any given genotype is determined by adding the effects of the two genes which make up the genotype. For example, if it is desired to know the reaction given by blood from an individual of genotype R^0r', one proceeds as follows:

	Reactions with Rh antisera			Reactions with Hr antisera	
	Anti-**Rh**₀	Anti-**rh′**	Anti-**rh″**	Anti-**hr′**	Anti-**hr″**
Gene R^0	+	−	−	+	+
Gene r'	−	+	−	−	+
By addition, genotype R^0r'	+	+	−	+	+

The phenotype name for blood giving positive reactions with all three Rh sera and with the two Hr sera is Rh_zRh_0 (cf. table 10). If tests are done with the three Rh antisera alone, and no Hr tests are done, the phenotype symbol Rh_z must be used instead. It should be emphasized that the results of the blood tests alone do not, as a rule, disclose the exact genotype of the individual being tested, so that the term "genotyping" for Rh-Hr typing is inaccurate. In fact, the genotype is only a theoretical concept based on the results of tests on the individual's blood together with similar serological tests on other members of his immediate family.

Frequency of gene R^Z: This is calculated most simply and reliably from the frequency of phenotype Rh_zRh_1. Of the three genotypes R^ZR^1, R^Zr', and R^1r^y corresponding to the phenotype Rh_zRh_1, the last two are so rare that they may be disregarded.

TABLE 11.—*The Rh-Hr Phenotypes and Genotypes*
Wiener's Multiple Allele Theory and Nomenclature

2 Rh Phenotypes			12 Rh Phenotypes					28 Rh-Hr Phenotypes					55 Genotypes*
Designations	Approximate frequencies in N.Y.C. whites (%)	Reaction with anti-Rh_0 (or anti-rhesus)	Designation†	Approximate frequencies in N.Y.C. whites (%)§	Anti-rh'	Anti-rh''	Anti-rh^w	Designation	Approximate frequencies in N.Y.C. whites (%)§	Anti-hr'	Anti-hr''	Anti-hr	
Rh negative	15	−	rh	14.4	−	−	−	rh	14.4	+	+	+	rr
			rh'	0.46‡	+	−	−	$rh'rh$	0.46	+	++	+	$r'r$
								$rh'rh'$	.0036	−	++	−	$r'r'$
			rh'^w	.004	+	−	+	rh'^wrh	.004	+	++	+	r'^wr
								rh'^wrh'	.00006	−	++	−	r'^wr' or $r'^wr'^w$
			rh''	0.38	−	+	−	$rh''rh$	0.38	++	+	+	$r''r$
								$rh''rh''$	.0025	++	−	−	$r''r''$
			rh_y	.01	+	+	−	$rh'rh''$	.006	+	+	−	$r'r''$
								rh_yrh	.008	+	+	+	r_yr
								rh_yrh'	.0001	−	+	−	r_yr'
								rh_yrh''	.0001	+	−	−	r_yr''
								rh_yrh_y	.000001	−	−	−	r_yr_y
			rh_y^w	.00005	+	+	+	rh'^wrh''	.00005	+	+	−	r'^wr''
								$rh_yrh'^w$	.000001	−	+	−	r'^wr_y

Rh	%	Rh₀	rh'	rhʷ	rh''	hr'	hr''	Rh₀	%	Genotypes
Rh positive	85	+								
Rh₀	2.1	+	−	−	−	+	+	Rh₀	2.1	R^0R^0 or R^0r
Rh₁	50.7	+	+	−	−	+	+	Rh₁rh	33.4	$R^1r, R^1R^0,$ or R^0r'
						−	+	Rh₁Rh₁	17.3	R^1R^1 or R^1r'
Rh₁ʷ	3.3	+	+	+	−	+	+	Rh₁ʷrh	1.6	$R^{1w}r, R^{1w}R^0,$ or $R^0r'^w$
						−	+	Rh₁ʷRh₁	1.7	$R^{1w}R^1, R^1r'^w, R^{1w}r',$ $R^{1w}R^{1w},$ or $R^{1w}r'^w$
Rh₂	14.6	+	−	−	+	+	+	Rh₂rh	12.2	$R^2r, R^2R^0,$ or R^0r''
						+	−	Rh₂Rh₂	2.4	R^2R^2 or R^2r''
Rhz	13.4	+	+	−	+	+	+	Rh₁Rh₂	12.9	$R^1R^2, R^1r'',$ or R^2r'
						+	+	Rhzrh	0.2	$R^Zr, R^ZR^0,$ or R^0r^y
						−	+	RhzRh₁	0.2	$R^ZR^1, R^Zr',$ or R^1r^y
						+	−	RhzRh₂	.07	$R^ZR^2, R^Zr'',$ or R^2r^y
						−	−	RhzRhz	.0004	R^ZR^Z or R^Zr^y
Rhzʷ	0.6	+	+	+	+	+	+	Rh₁ʷRh₂	0.6	$R^{1w}R^2, R^{1w}r'',$ or $R^2r'^w$
						−	+	RhzʷRh₁	.008	$R^{1w}R^Z, R^{1w}r^y,$ or $R^Zr'^w$

* This table does not include genes R^{zw} and r^{yw}, which appear to be very rare.

† In this table Rh_1 is used as a short designation for Rh'_0; Rh_2 is short for Rh''_0; rh_y is short for rh'''; and Rh_Z is short for Rh'''_0.

‡ The reduction in the frequency of type rh' as compared with that given in earlier charts can be attributed to recognition of bloods of type Rh_1 (containing Rh_0 variant), which are now included in type Rh_1 instead of rh'. The agglutinogens Rh_0, Rh_1, and Rh_2, and their corresponding genes R^0, R^1, and R^2, are not given here, because this would serve unnecessarily to complicate the chart, by increasing the number of possible genotypes to 91. Also, no attempt is made to include certain rare exceptional bloods, such as those lacking both factors rh' and hr', and/or lacking both rh'' and hr'', etc.

§ Based on the estimated gene frequencies, $r = 0.38$, $r' = .006$, $r'' = .005$, $r^y = .0001$, $r'^w = .00005$, $R^0 = .027$, $R^1 = 0.41$, $R^2 = 0.15$, $R^Z = .002$, and $R^{1w} = .02$.

Therefore, the frequency of gene R^Z can be estimated simply by dividing the frequency of phenotype $Rh_Z Rh_1$ by twice the frequency of gene R^1 (*cf.* tables 8 and 11). The rare gene R^Z has its highest frequency among Mongoloids.

Frequency of gene r^y: This can be estimated from the frequency of the phenotype $rh_y rh$, corresponding to which there are two possible genotypes $r'r''$ and $r^y r$. From family studies (*cf.* table 9) it appears that about half of type $rh_y rh$ Caucasoids are of genotype $r'r''$ and about half genotype $r^y r$. Therefore, the frequency of gene r^y equals about half the frequency of phenotype $rh_y rh$ divided by twice the frequency of gene r (*cf.* tables 8 and 11).

Statistical test of the theory of multiple alleles: The frequencies of the genes r, r'', r'', R^0, R^1, and R^2 can be calculated by means of the square root formulae given on page 33, while r^y and R^Z are estimated by the methods given above. The theory of multiple alleles requires that the sum of these calculated frequencies equals 100 per cent. Moreover, since factors **rh'** and **hr'** are reciprocally related, and factors **rh''** and **hr''** are similarly reciprocally related, the following additional relationships should hold:

$$\sqrt{rh'-} + \sqrt{hr'-} = 100 \text{ per cent} \qquad (7)$$
$$\sqrt{rh''-} + \sqrt{hr''-} = 100 \text{ per cent} \qquad (8)$$

In table 12, R. R. Race's excellent data on the distribution of the Rh-Hr types in London have been subjected to statistical analysis, and it can be seen that they satisfy the requirements of the genetic theory. The same has proved to be true of all other populations subjected to this statistical test.

Factor hr: A blood factor detected by the serum designated anti-**hr** and which is shared by agglutinogen rh and Rh_0 (determined by the genes r and R^0, respectively), but not by the other Rh-Hr agglutinogens. Thus, an individual carrying either of the genes r or R^0, or both genes, will be positive for factor **hr**, while all other individuals will be negative (*cf.* table 8). The main value of anti-**hr** serum is for testing bloods from individuals of phenotypes $Rh_Z Rh_0$ and $rh_y rh$, each of which phenotype is subdivided by its reaction with anti-**hr** serum. In this way it is possible to determine, for example, whether an individual of phenotype $Rh_Z Rh_0$ belongs to the phenotype

TABLE 12.—*Statistical Analysis of R. R. Race's Data on the Distribution of the Rh-Hr Types in London*

Rh-Hr Phenotypes	Number	Per Cent
rh	170	15.84
rh'rh'	0	0
rh'rh	10	0.93
rh''rh''	0	0
rh''rh	7	0.65
rh_yrh rh_yrh' rh_yrh'' rh_yrh_y	0	0
Rh_0	19	1.77
Rh_1Rh_1	190	17.71
Rh_1rh	363	33.83
Rh_2Rh_2	29	2.70
Rh_2rh	137	12.77
Rh_zRh_0	144	13.42
Rh_zRh_1	4	0.37
Rh_zRh_2 Rh_zRh_z	0	0

$r = 39.80; r' = 1.15; r'' = 0.81; R^0 = 2.19; R^1 = 40.57; R^2 = 15.28; R^Z = 0.44;$
thus $\Sigma R = 100.24.$

$\sqrt{(rh'-)} + \sqrt{(hr'-)} = 100.59$ per cent; $\sqrt{(rh''-)} + \sqrt{(hr''-)} = 100.11$ per cent.

Rh_1Rh_2 comprising the three genotypes R^1R^2, R^1r'', and R^2r' (hr negative) or to phenotype Rh_zrh comprising the three genotypes R^Zr, R^ZR^0, and R^0r^y (hr positive), as shown in table 11. Such information may prove useful in medicolegal cases of disputed paternity, as well as in clinical work. In all other cases, anti-hr serum gives negative reactions when and only when anti-hr' and/or anti-hr'' serum gives a negative reaction. In table 8 are listed eight of the more important allelic genes, the so-called standard Rh-Hr genes, showing their relationship to factor hr as well as to other Rh-Hr blood factors.

Rh variants: Occasionally blood specimens are encountered which give weak or intermediate reactions with one or more of the Rh-Hr antisera, demonstrating the existence of variants of the Rh-Hr factors. Of these the most important are the variants of the **Rh₀** factor (designated as factor $\Re h_0$). The so-called $\Re h_0$ actually comprises a series of related factors, which according to their reactions are designated as "high-grade" or "low-grade" variants. Factor $\Re h_0$ can occur in the absence of factors **rh′** and **rh″** (type $\Re h_0$), or in association with factor **rh′** but not **rh″** (type $\Re h_1$), or in association with **rh″** but not **rh′** (type $\Re h_2$), or in association with both factors **rh′** and **rh″** (type $\Re h_Z$). Thus, there are four different diagnoses to be made: between type rh and type $\Re h_0$, between type rh′ and type $\Re h_1$, between type rh″ and type $\Re h_2$, and between type rh_y and type $\Re h_Z$. Rh₀ variants are rare and occur most frequently among Negroes as the phenotype $\Re h_0$. In Caucasians, factor $\Re h_0$ occurs most often in association with factor **rh′**, and as many as half of the specimens originally typed as type rh′ are now known to belong to type $\Re h_1$. The most reliable way of recognizing factor $\Re h_0$ is by the negative or doubtful reactions with anti-$\Re h_0$ agglutinating serum in the test tube, while distinct positive reactions occur by the slide or tube conglutination test, or the proteolytic enzyme method, and especially by the anti-globulin method in tests with appropriate anti-**Rh₀** conglutinating serum. The four agglutinogens $\Re h_0$, $\Re h_1$, $\Re h_2$, and $\Re h_Z$ appear to be inherited by corresponding allelic genes $\Re^0$, $\Re^1$, $\Re^2$, and $\Re^Z$, thus increasing further the Rh series of allelic genes.

Practical significance of the Rh₀ variants: Blood having an Rh₀ variant may be typed as Rh negative or Rh positive, depending on the anti-**Rh₀** serum and technic used, and this may lead to confusion unless the true situation is recognized. Donors with an $\Re h_0$ factor should be classified as Rh positive, because injection of such blood into an Rh-negative recipient can lead to **Rh₀** sensitization, though less readily than injections of "standard" Rh-positive blood. On the other hand, individuals who are $\Re h_0$ positive may occasionally produce antibodies resembling anti-**Rh₀** in specificity. The reason for this appears to be that blood having an Rh₀ variant frequently lacks one or more of the associated factors, **Rh^A**, **Rh^B**, **Rh^C**, **Rh^D**, etc. Since such persons can be sensitized to the factor missing from their blood, they may produce anti-**Rh^A**, anti-**Rh^B**, etc., as the case may be, which resemble anti-**Rh₀** in specificity (*cf.* page 31). Therefore, when $\Re h_0$-positive individuals are recipients, they should preferably be treated as Rh-negative to avoid sensitization, and if they are already sensitized, obviously, transfusions of unselected Rh-positive blood could cause a hemolytic reaction.

Types $\overline{\overline{R}}h_0$ and $\overline{\overline{R}}h^w$: Two extremely rare phenotypes which share the property of lacking both factor pairs **rh'-hr'** and **rh''-hr''**, as indicated by the use of a double bar above the R of the phenotype symbol. The existence of such bloods demonstrates that the reciprocal relationship between factor **rh'** and **hr'** and between **rh''** and **hr''** is not absolute. The agglutinogens $\overline{\overline{R}}h_0$ and $\overline{\overline{R}}h^w$ also share the property of high reactivity with anti-**Rh**$_0$ sera, so that the blood cells may be clumped by anti-**rh'** and anti-**rh''** reagents containing **Rh**$_0$ blocking antibody (*cf.* page 22) even when the tests are done in saline media. Persons who belong to phenotypes $\overline{\overline{R}}h_0$ and $\overline{\overline{R}}h^w$ appear to be easily sensitized by transfusion or pregnancy, and may produce anti-**rh'**, anti-**hr'**, anti-**rh''**, and anti-**hr''**, or combinations of these. As a rule, however, they form an antibody designated anti-**Hr**, which reacts with all bloods except those of phenotypes $\overline{\overline{R}}h_0$ and $\overline{\overline{R}}h^w$. Obviously, anti-**Hr** will therefore simulate the reactions of anti-**rh'** and anti-**hr'** in combination, or anti-**rh''** and anti-**hr''** in combination. However, it has been proved by absorption studies that a single antibody, specific for a unit blood factor, **Hr**, is involved in these reactions. The transfusion of such sensitized persons and of erythroblastotic babies in these rare circumstances poses a serious problem, which has only been solved with the aid of blood bank clearing houses where lists of individuals of rare blood types are kept.

To account for agglutinogens $\overline{\overline{R}}h_0$ and $\overline{\overline{R}}h^w$, two corresponding allelic genes $\overline{\overline{R}}^0$ and $\overline{\overline{R}}^w$ have been postulated, and the existence of these genes has been confirmed by family studies. Obviously, individuals of type $\overline{\overline{R}}h_0$ must be of genotype $\overline{\overline{R}}^0\overline{\overline{R}}^0$, while persons of type $\overline{\overline{R}}h^w$ are of genotype $\overline{\overline{R}}^w\overline{\overline{R}}^w$. Heterozygous individuals carrying the gene $\overline{\overline{R}}^0$ may give rise to exceptions to the eight-gene theory of the inheritance of the Rh-Hr blood types; e.g., an individual of phenotype Rh$_1$Rh$_1$ could have a type Rh$_0$ child, if instead of genotype R^1R^1 or R^1r' the parent was actually of genotype $R^1\overline{\overline{R}}^0$ and his child of genotype $\overline{\overline{R}}^0r$ or $R^0\overline{\overline{R}}^0$.

Type $\overline{R}h_0$: Blood having the factors **Rh**$_0$ and **hr'**, but lacking **rh'** and both factors of the contrasting pair **rh''-hr''**, as indicated by the single bar above the R in the symbol. This type of blood may rarely

TABLE 13.—*The Rh-Hr Series of Allelic Genes, the Rh-Hr Agglutinogens, and Their Blood Factors*

Gene Symbol	Agglutinogen Symbol	1 Rh_0	2 rh'	3 rh^{w1}	4 rh''	5 rh^{w2}	6 hr'	7 hr''	8 hr	9 Rh^A	10 Rh^B	11 Rh^C	12 Rh^D	13 rh^x	14 rh_i	15 rh^G	16 Hr	17 hr^S	18 hr^V	19 hr^N
1. r	rh	−	−	−	−	−	+	+	+	−	−	−	−	−	−	−	+	+	−	−
2. r'	rh'	−	+	−	−	−	−	+	−	−	−	−	−	−	+	+	+	+	−	−
3. r^w	rh^w	−	+	+	−	−	−	+	−	−	−	−	−	−	+	+	+	+	−	−
4. r''	rh''	−	−	−	+	−	+	−	−	−	−	−	−	−	−	−	+	−	−	−
5. r^y	rh_y	−	+	−	+	−	−	−	−	−	−	−	−	−	−	+	+	−	−	−
6. R^0	Rh_0	+	−	−	−	−	+	+	+	+	+	+	+	−	−	+	+	+	−	−
7. R^1	Rh_1	+	+	−	−	−	−	+	−	+	+	+	+	−	+	+	+	+	−	−
8. R^{1w}	Rh_1^w	+	+	+	−	−	−	+	−	+	+	+	+	−	+	+	+	+	−	−
9. R^2	Rh_2	+	−	−	+	−	+	−	−	+	+	+	+	−	−	+	+	−	−	−
10. R^z	Rh_z	+	+	−	+	−	−	−	−	+	+	+	+	−	−	+	+	−	−	−
11. $\Re^0$	$\Re h_0$	±	−	−	−	−	+	+	+	±	±	±	±	−	−	+	+	+	−	−
12. $\Re^1$	$\Re h_1$	±	+	−	−	−	−	+	−	±	±	±	±	−	+	+	+	+	−	−
13. $\Re^2$	$\Re h_2$	±	−	−	+	−	+	−	−	±	±	±	±	−	−	+	+	−	−	−

No.	Gene	Rh type	1	2	3	4	5	6	7	8	9	10	11	12	13	14	15	16	17	18	19
14	$\parallel R^0$	$\parallel Rh_0$	−	−	−	−	+	−	−	+	+	+	+	−	−	−	−	−	−	−	+
15	$\parallel R^w$	$\parallel Rh^w$	−	−	−	−	+	−	−	+	+	+	+	−	−	−	−	−	+	−	+
16	R^0	Rh_0	−	−	−	−	+	−	−	+	+	+	+	+	−	+	−	−	−	−	+
17	R^0	Rh_0	−	−	−	−	+	−	−	+	+	+	+	+	+	+	−	−	−	−	+
18	r	rh	−	−	−	−	−	−	−	−	−	−	−	−	−	−	−	−	−	−	−
19	R^{1x}	Rh_1^x	−	−	+	+	+	+	+	+	+	+	+	−	+	−	−	−	−	+	+
20	R^{2w}	Rh_2^w	−	−	−	+	+	−	−	+	+	+	+	−	−	+	+	+	−	−	+
21	r^v	rh^v	+	+	+	+	−	−	−	−	−	−	−	+	+	+	−	−	−	−	−
22	R^{0v}	Rh_0^v	+	+	+	+	+	−	−	+	+	+	+	+	+	+	−	−	−	−	+
23	r'^N	rh'^N	+	−	+	+	+	−	−	−	−	−	−	+	+	+	−	−	−	+	−
24	R^{1ab}	Rh_1^{ab}	−	−	+	+	+	+	−	+	+	−	−	−	+	−	−	−	−	+	+
25	R^{2b}	Rh_2^b	−	−	−	+	+	−	−	+	+	−	+	−	−	+	−	+	−	−	+
26	$\Re^{2c}$	$\Re h_2^c$	−	−	−	+	+	−	−	+	−	+	+	−	−	+	−	+	−	−	+
27	R^{0d}	Rh_0^d	−	−	+	+	+	−	−	−	+	+	+	+	+	+	−	−	−	−	+
28	r^G	rh^G	−	−	−	+	+	−	−	−	−	−	−	−	+	−	−	−	−	−	−

be found among Negroids, where it will give rise to apparent contradictions to the genetic theory. Thus, a mother of phenotype Rh_2Rh_2 could have a child of phenotype Rh_0 if the parent is of genotype $R^2\overline{R}^0$ and the child of genotype $R^0\overline{R}^0$. Sensitized individuals of type Rh_0 may produce antibodies resembling anti-**Hr** in specificity. It is of interest that a related Rh-Hr type ($\overline{Rh}_0{}^{Ch}$) appears to be prevalent among chimpanzees, whose bloods regularly have factors Rh_0 and **hr′**, but lack **rh′**, **rh″**, and **hr″**.

Type $\overline{rh}$: An extremely rare type of blood, lacking all of the known Rh-Hr blood factors. So far only a single individual, an Australian aborigine, has been found of this type.

Factor hr^S: A factor almost regularly associated with factor **hr″**. Blood having **hr″** without hr^S does occur rarely, however, especially among Negroids. This is indicated by placing a caret above the R in the symbol. Because of the similarity of the reactions, anti-hr^S has been confused with anti-**hr″**, and many such antisera contain both antibodies. The unwitting use of anti-hr^S in place of anti-**hr″** can give rise to apparent contradictions to the genetic theory, e.g., a mother of genotype $R^2\hat{R}^0$ may be mistyped as phenotype Rh_2Rh_2 (instead of $Rh_2\hat{R}h_0$) causing confusion should her child be type Rh_0 (genotype $\hat{R}^0r$ or $R^0\hat{R}^0$).

Series of Rh-Hr allelic genes: It is evident that as more Rh-Hr factors are found, a continually increasing number of Rh-Hr phenotypes are being distinguished, increasing in turn the number of known Rh-Hr allelic genes. In fact, the number already demonstrated to exist is too great to be given in a simple table. A list of the more important known genes is given in table 13 for purposes of reference.

CHAPTER IV

Erythroblastosis Fetalis

Erythroblastosis fetalis; hemolytic disease of the newborn:
A disease of the newborn caused by isosensitization of the expectant mother to an agglutinogen present in the red cells of the fetus but absent in her own blood cells. The isoantibodies which are produced by the mother pass across the placental barrier into the circulation of the fetus in utero where they combine with and coat the red cells of the fetus. The isoantibody most commonly responsible for erythroblastosis fetalis is anti-Rh_0, as was first demonstrated by Levine et al. Depending primarily on the titer and the avidity of the maternal antibodies, the disease may manifest itself as an hydropic stillbirth, or if the baby is born alive he may exhibit various degrees of icterus and anemia, sometimes severe enough to cause death in the newborn period. In the less common cases of erythroblastosis where the mother is Rh_0 positive, the disease may result from isosensitization to one of the Hr factors, most often **hr′**, or to factors **rh′**, **rh″**, or **rh**^{w}, to the **A** or **B** factors (e.g., mother group O, and baby group A or B), or rarely to sensitization to a factor of some other blood group system, notably **K** (Kell), or even to sensitization to combinations of two or more blood factors.

Antenatal case finding: The program designed to anticipate the occurrence of erythroblastosis in the as yet unborn infant. By the use of blood tests alone, it is, as a rule, possible to predict the probable occurrence of the disease, so that early delivery can be carried out if necessary, and preparations made for prompt treatment of the affected infant, if he is live born. Every expectant mother should be tested for the Rh_0 factor, and if Rh negative, the husband's blood is typed. If the husband is also Rh negative, no further tests need be done, because all the children will be Rh negative. If he is Rh positive, tests for Rh antibodies should be carried out on the expectant mother's serum (*cf.* page 22). If the expectant Rh-negative mother is sensitized, the Rh antibodies should be titrated by all the standard technics (*cf.* Chapter II), and, if possible, complete Rh-Hr typing of the husband and any living children carried out in an attempt to predict the expected baby's Rh type. If the husband is homozygous Rh positive, the expected baby will be Rh positive and almost surely affected if the mother is sensitized; if the husband is heterozygous Rh positive, there is a 50 per cent chance of an Rh-negative baby who will not be harmed by the maternal antibodies. A significant rise in titer during the course of a pregnancy can be taken as proof that the expected baby is Rh positive, and therefore probably affected by the disease.

Such a routine will detect more than 90 per cent of cases of erythroblastosis, except those due to A-B-O incompatibility, before birth. Most of the remaining cases luckily tend to be less severe, and can be generally diagnosed shortly after birth and proper treatment instituted.

Cases of erythroblastosis due to other factors such as **hr'** can be anticipated antenatally by screening the sera of Rh-positive as well as Rh-negative expectant mothers for abnormal antibodies against a suitable panel of cells, preferably by the ficinated cell or a comparable technic.

Titer of Rh antibodies in expectant mother's serum: The concentration of Rh antibodies in the maternal serum, generally expressed in units (*cf.* page 26). This is one of the most important factors affecting the prognosis of the erythroblastotic infant, as shown by the close correlation between Rh antibody titer and stillbirth rate (*cf.* table 14). However, the correlation between antibody titer and severity is by no means absolute, since, for example, babies have developed severe jaundice despite the presence of only mild sensitization, while other babies have remained normal clinically in the presence of a high maternal titer of incompatible antibodies, sufficient to produce maximal coating of their red cells and a high titer of free antibodies in the baby's own serum.

Molecular size of antibody: Another important factor affecting prognosis, as has been shown by Wiener. Bivalent antibodies (or agglutinins) which are of greater molecular size (19S) do not traverse the intact placental barrier and therefore cannot harm the Rh-positive baby; univalent antibodies (7S), on the other hand, readily

TABLE 14.—*Relationship Between Antibody Titer and Stillbirth Rate*

Titer* of Rh Antibodies (units)	Total Number of Fetuses and Babies		Stillbirths	
	Rh positive	Rh negative	Number	Per cent
0	234	104	4	1.2
0†	6	—	0	0
less than 4	49	—	3	6.1
up to 16	50	—	6	12.0
up to 64	63	—	16	25.4
up to 256	18	—	8	44.4
up to 1024	2	—	2	100.0
1 to 1000	—	23	0	0

* By albumin-plasma conglutination method.
† But positive by the enzyme technique.
(Wiener, A. S., Nappi, R., and Gordon, E. B.: Am. J. Obst. & Gynec. *63:* 6, 1952.)

pass through the placenta and coat the baby's red cells, causing intravascular hemolysis and/or clumping (*cf.* table 5). Almost all sensitized persons produce both forms of antibody, though one form or the other may predominate. When **Rh₀** agglutinins in the maternal serum are present in high titer, it is difficult to determine the titer of the more important univalent antibodies. If such sera are heated for an hour at 60 C. to destroy the heat labile bivalent antibodies (*cf.* table 5), any univalent antibodies which may be present will then be readily demonstrable. Despite the presence of high-titered Rh agglutinins, the prognosis for the newborn baby is generally good, so long as the tests show only a small quantity of univalent antibodies. When the sensitized mother has an Rh-negative baby, the titer of the univalent Rh antibodies is almost invariably the same in the mother and in the baby, but bivalent antibodies are never found in the newborn baby's blood. By following the titer of the passively acquired univalent antibodies in Rh-negative babies, it has been found that the half-life of such antibodies is 30 to 35 days.

Avidity of antibodies: The degree of affinity between an antibody and the corresponding antigen or blood factor. Poorly adapted antibodies do not combine firmly with their antigens and are readily eluted. Antibodies of a given specificity, such as **Rh**$_0$, may vary in avidity, while some cases of mild disease despite high antibody titer may be due to low avidity (*cf.* table 15). (In the counterpart of the latter situation, the mother's serum contains **Rh**$_0$ antibodies of high avidity, but the baby's cells contain blood factor $\mathfrak{Rh}_0$ instead of **Rh**$_0$. Here again the clinical manifestations are generally mild.) As in the case of antibody titer, the correlation between avidity and severity is a statistical one and is by no means absolute.

TABLE 15.—*Avidity of Rh Antibodies and Prognosis*

Type of Rh$_0$ Antibody*	Where Found	Titer (units) by Method of				
		Agglutination in saline mediums	Blocking test	Albumin-plasma conglutination	Antiglobulin	Enzyme-treated cells (ficin or papain)
High avidity	Hyperimmunized male donors Women having repeated stillbirths Patients sensitized by multiple transfusions. Severe hemolytic reactions	0	10	500	500	500
Average avidity	Typical severe cases of erythroblastosis	0	1	30	150	300
Low avidity	Subclinical cases of erythroblastosis, or baby unaffected	0	0	0	2	200
Mixture Rh agglutinin and low avidity univalent Rh antibody	Baby unaffected though Rh positive	20	—	20	49	200

* Some sera contain mixtures of Rh antibodies of different avidities as can be shown by absorption experiments.

Undefined constitutional factors in the baby: Agents other than serological, and probably genetic, which are postulated to play a role in the pathogenesis of the disease. Because the correlation between antibody titer and/or avidity and the severity of the disease is not absolute, it is evident that other factors influence the course of the disease. Of particular significance in this regard are observations which have been made on certain pairs of fraternal twins who are of the same sex and have identical serological findings, but who exhibit quite different clinical manifestations.

Role of blood injections: Rh hemolytic disease only infrequently affects the first born baby, except in cases where the mother has been sensitized by an intramuscular or intravenous injection of blood, or of improperly prepared plasma or serum containing red cell stromata. At one time, newborn babies and children were given intramuscular injections of untyped blood for treatment of hemorrhagic manifestations, or for prophylaxis of certain contagious diseases, and young Rh-negative girls or women, either through error or ignorance, were transfused with Rh-positive blood, especially in emergency situations. The sensitization resulting from such procedures have affected the first-born Rh-positive baby, who not infrequently was stillborn, or, if born alive, was severely erythroblastotic. Nowadays, of course, no Rh-negative girl or woman of childbearing age, or any other Rh-negative person, is deliberately injected with Rh-positive blood except under the most unusual circumstances. Rh sensitization resulting from such injections has been the cause of law suits, and in some cases there have been substantial awards for medical liability.

Role of parity: Each incompatible pregnancy carries with it the opportunity of isosensitization of the mother. The normal placenta is impervious to red cells, but indirect evidence obtained by following the course of antibody titers during pregnancy indicates that in about one out of three pregnancies, and in about one out of three deliveries, whether vaginal or Cesarean, some fetal red cells enter the maternal circulation and further sensitize her. Naturally, the chance of sensitization increases with each pregnancy and a calculation based on the experience with deliberately injected donors shows a reasonable agreement between the expected frequency of sensitization and that actually observed (*cf.* table 16). It should be pointed out that although Rh sensitization does not cause early abortions, each

TABLE 16.—*Frequency of Rh Sensitization in Relation to Parity*

Parity	McLean et al. (U.S.A.)			Nevanlinna and Vainio (Finland)		
	Total number of Rh-negative mothers	Sensitized mothers		Total number of Rh-negative mothers	Sensitized mothers	
		Number	Per cent		Number	Per cent
i	486	2	0.4	4,153	10	0.2
ii	306	17	5.3	3,298	89	2.7
iii	149	23	15.4	1,992	115	5.8
iv	77	17	22.1	1,186	75	6.3
v	24	8	33.3	615	48	7.8
vi or more	6	3	50.0	703	72	10.2
Totals	1,048	70	6.7	11,947	409	3.4

abortion constitutes another opportunity to bring about such sensitization. Although accurate data are not available it seems that abnormal pregnancies such as ectopic gestation and placenta previa, ablatio placentae, etc., are somewhat more apt to bring about sensitization than normal pregnancies.

Heterospecific and homospecific pregnancies: When the baby's A-B-O blood group is incompatible with the mother's (e.g., baby group A, mother group O), the pregnancy is said to be heterospecific, while if the baby's blood group is compatible (e.g., baby group O, mother group A), the pregnancy is said to be homospecific. Levine pointed out that in families with erythroblastotic babies due to Rh incompatibility, the husband's A-B-O blood group is compatible with that of the mother more often than in the general population (*cf.* table 17). Although this has been ascribed to competition between the A-B and Rh antigens, the more likely explanation is that A-B-O incompatible fetal blood entering the maternal circulation is immediately lysed and eliminated, thus reducing the opportunity for sensitization to the Rh factor to develop. Thus an Rh-negative mother is less apt to become sensitized if her husband is of an incompatible A-B-O group than if he is of a compatible group.

Role of zygosity of the husband: If the husband is homozygous with respect to the Rh_0 factor, every child must be Rh_0 positive, so that the chance of sensitization by pregnancy will be greater than

TABLE 17.—*Relative Frequency of Compatible and Incompatible Matings in Relation to the Clinical Manifestations in the Fetus and Newborn*

Clinical Manifestation	Total Number of Cases	Compatible		Incompatible	
		Number	Per cent	Number	Per cent
Unexplained neonatal jaundice or anemia...................	94	19	20.2	75	79.8
Two or more abortions..........	89	43	47.3	46	52.7
Erythroblastosis due to Rh sensitization......................	282	232	82.2	50	17.8
Miscellaneous*.................	377	238	63.3	139	36.7
Theoretical distribution in random matings................	—	—	65	—	35

(Wiener, A. S., Wexler, I. B., and Hurst, J. G.: Blood *4:* 1014, 1949.)

* These comprise all normal and abnormal infants not included in the other categories.

when the husband is heterozygous. Moreover, once sensitization is established, if the husband is heterozygous, there would be a fifty per cent chance of the baby being Rh negative and therefore not affected by the maternal isoantibodies. Anti-**Hr**$_0$ serum which could establish the zygosity of the husband with certainty has not been found, but an approximation can be made with the aid of anti-**hr'** and anti-**hr''** sera. For example, a type Rh$_1$Rh$_1$ husband would most frequently be homozygous (genotype R^1R^1) though occasionally he will prove to be heterozygous (genotype R^1r') for blood factor **Rh**$_0$. Similarly, a type Rh$_1$rh husband would most frequently be heterozygous (genotype R^1r), though less frequently he may prove to be homozygous (genotype R^1R^0) for blood factor **Rh**$_0$. A more precise diagnosis of zygosity may be possible from family studies, and is of value for prognostic purposes.

Salk vaccine and maternal sensitization: Because polio vaccine is prepared by culturing the polio virus on rhesus monkey kidney tissue, the question has been raised whether administration of the vaccine to expectant Rh-negative mothers might sensitize them to the Rh factor. Experimental inoculation of already sensitized Rh-negative persons with Salk vaccine produced no rise in Rh antibody titer, even though subsequent injections of Rh-positive blood in the same individuals stimulated a rise in titer. This is evidence that injection of Salk vaccine does not sensitize Rh-negative individuals to the Rh factor.

Time and route of delivery: These are other factors affecting the prognosis in erythroblastosis fetalis. Obviously the longer the fetus is exposed to the maternal antibodies, the greater is the chance that the baby may be severely affected. Therefore, when the indication exists, delivery should be accomplished 2 to 3 weeks before term. Since most sensitized women are multipara, induction of labor can generally be carried out with relative ease. When setting the date of delivery, the dangers of prematurity should be weighed against the dangers of prolonged exposure to the maternal antibodies, since premature infants with their poorly developed enzyme systems are particularly susceptible to the harmful effects of the disease, as well as to the handling entailed in carrying out an exchange transfusion. It is good practice to consult with the obstetrician for an estimate of the probable weight and maturity of the expected infant, and to take into account all of the factors involved before delivery is induced. Erythroblastosis fetalis *per se* is not an indication for Cesarean section, but this must be done, of course, when an obstetric indication exists. Clearly, labor should not be induced early if there is a reasonable chance that the baby will be Rh negative (*cf.* Zygosity and Anamnestic Reactions).

Blood group loci: The points on the discoplasm (or stroma of the erythrocyte) at which the blood group agglutinogens are situated. There are separate loci for every blood group system, and the agglutinogens of each system are thought of as being repeated more or less regularly on the surface of the red cells (*cf.* figure 2). The A-B-O loci are most numerous, which may explain in part why **A** and **B** antibodies are capable (in the presence of complement) of producing hemolysis in in vitro tests despite their relatively low avidity. The Rh-Hr loci are less numerous, so that despite the high avidity of such antibodies, hemolysis does not occur in the in vitro tests. In fact, in some erythroblastotic babies the hemoglobin concentration falls only very gradually even though the cells are coated with Rh antibodies, and some of these babies may recover without any treatment. Loci of other blood group systems such as Kell and Duffy, are even less numerous than Rh, so that **K** and **F** antibodies would not be expected to give rise to severe erythroblastosis even when they are of high titer and avidity.

Direct antiglobulin test; direct Coombs' test: A test for coating or sensitization of the red cells by **Rh**$_0$ or other antibodies; a test generally pathognomonic for typical erythroblastosis fetalis. This important delicate test is performed as follows. The red cells of the baby are washed three or four times with a large excess of saline solution in order to remove all but the minutest traces of serum proteins, and then resuspended to make a 2 to 4 per cent suspension. One drop of the washed cells is mixed with a drop of antihuman globulin serum in a small tube, and the mixture centrifuged at 500 rpm for 1 minute, the tube shaken and then examined for clumping. Positive reactions occur almost invariably in typical erythroblastosis caused by Rh or Hr sensitization. In the disease caused by **A** or **B** sensitization, the reaction is characteristically negative or very weak, although in rare cases it may be quite distinct (*cf.* page 68). In instances of **Kell** sensitization or in mild cases of **Rh**$_0$ sensitization, the reactions are generally weaker, apparently due to the lower number of antigenic loci coated by antibodies. In occasional instances of erythroblastosis, the maternal antibodies, though of high titer by the proteolytic enzyme technic, may not react or hardly react by the antiglobulin method. In such cases, the direct Coombs' test may be negative.

Direct conglutination test (Wiener): Coating of red cells by Rh antibodies can also be demonstrated by suspending the infant's cells in plasma, or, better, in albumin-plasma mixtures, or in acacia, whereupon clumping by conglutination results. The direct conglutination test is somewhat less sensitive than the direct antiglobulin test, so that it is generally positive only in more severely affected babies.

Direct blocking test (Wiener): Cells which are completely coated with **Rh**$_0$ blocking antibodies, such as occurs in the case of **Rh**$_0$-positive babies of strongly sensitized women, may be completely blocked. Such cells have been incorrectly typed as Rh negative, especially when the tests are carried out by the tube agglutination method.

Quantitative direct antiglobulin test (Wiener): A test to determine the degree of coating of red cells by antibodies. To carry out the test, the cells of the erythroblastotic baby are washed four times with an excess of saline solution, and an anti-human globulin serum is then titrated against the washed cells. At the same time, the antiglobulin serum is titrated against Rh-positive cells which have been maximally sensitized with Rh_0 univalent antiserum and then washed with saline solution. The degree of coating in per cent is calculated by dividing the titer of the antiglobulin serum for the baby's cells by its titer for maximally sensitized Rh-positive cells, and multiplying by 100. As might be expected, the severity of the manifestations in the erythroblastotic infant is correlated with the degree of coating of the red cells.

By applying this method to red cells maximally coated with **K** and **F** antibodies, it has been found that there are only about one-fourth as many **K** loci and one-tenth as many **F** loci as there are Rh-Hr loci on the red cell surface.

Complement and conglutinin: The concentration of conglutinin and complement in the fetus in utero is lower than in the adult, in parallel with the lower concentration of serum proteins. After birth, possibly as the result of dehydration, the concentration increases during the first few days of life, though not to the adult level. This may be the reason why, in many babies, the birth itself, whether spontaneous or induced, appears to initiate or aggravate the disease process. While the idea of the role of fetal complement and conglutinin appears attractive, tests on babies with marked serological findings, but without clinical evidence of disease, have disclosed no abnormality in complement or conglutinin concentration in the serum.

Rh antigen in tissue and body fluid: Carefully controlled experiments have failed to disclose the presence of the Rh antigen outside the red cells. Reports in the literature to the contrary are probably due to artifacts. There is no convincing evidence to support the idea that Rh antibodies cause brain and liver damage, or damage to any other tissue, by direct action of the antibodies on the tissue cells; instead, Wiener believes that the lesions encountered in the erythroblastotic infant are due, at least in part, to intravascular conglutination of red cells with blocking of the circulation.

Erythroblastemia: The presence of nucleated red blood cells in the blood stream. It is from this manifestation that the disease acquired its name. In the most severe cases of erythroblastosis the blood smear may be so heavily laden with erythroblasts as to present a superficial resemblance to leukemia. With improved diagnostic methods for determining Rh sensitization, it has become clear that erythroblastemia is not an essential feature of the disease and may even be entirely absent. Nevertheless, it is still convenient to use the term erythroblastosis fetalis for the syndrome resulting from isosensitization. Newborn infants characteristically respond to stress by pouring out erythroblasts from the bone marrow, particularly in those conditions associated with anemia, so that the finding of excessive numbers of these cells in the peripheral blood of a neonate is by no means pathognomonic of erythroblastosis fetalis.

Anemia: Another common manifestation of erythroblastosis fetalis. This is thought to be the result of the hemolytic effect of the Rh antibodies on the infant's Rh-positive red cells. As with erythroblastemia, anemia is most marked in the most severely affected infants. The normal hemoglobin concentration as determined on the cord blood averages 16.6 Gm. per cent, while the peripheral blood hemoglobin concentration will depend upon the time that the cord is clamped, being higher if the cord is clamped late. As far as the outcome of the disease is concerned, early or late clamping of the cord appears to be of no consequence. It is important to note that anemia with little or no jaundice is an infrequent finding in erythroblastosis fetalis, and in an infant presenting this combination of signs, the possibility of fetal blood loss by transplacental feto-maternal transfusion must be considered. This, of course, is the mechanism of maternal sensitization, and while ordinarily the amount of fetal blood loss is insignificant, in rare cases it may be large enough to cause the death of the infant.

Hepatosplenomegaly: Enlargement of the liver and the spleen, nearly always found in the more severely affected infants. Microscopic examination of these organs shows that the enlargement is due to nests of erythropoietic tissue. When recovery takes place the organs return to their normal size, without scarring.

Hemorrhage: A manifestation occasionally encountered in erythroblastosis fetalis, which may present as multiple petechiae or as ecchymoses accompanied by oozing of blood from the nose and mouth. The latter is a reflection of intrapulmonary bleeding and is of grave prognostic significance. The antigen-antibody reaction is believed to initiate hemorrhage in the erythroblastotic baby by reducing the platelet count and depleting the blood of fibrinogen, and perhaps also by producing intravascular conglutination. This manifestation may possibly be related to the Schwartzmann phenomenon.

Hyperbilirubinemia: An increase in the concentration of bilirubin in the blood serum; one of the major manifestations of erythroblastosis fetalis. The bilirubin concentration in the umbilical cord serum of normal babies ranges up to 2.5 mg. per cent, as compared with about 0.5 mg. per cent in the normal older child or adult. During the first 4 days of life, an evanescent mild hyperbilirubinemia occurs in most normal full-term infants, reflecting the incapacity of the newborn baby's liver (or other organs) to conjugate bilirubin. In premature infants, the peak concentrations of serum bilirubin are generally higher, with the highest values occurring in the more premature babies. In erythroblastosis fetalis, the degree of hyperbilirubinemia can become extreme, and in the most severely affected infants, concentrations as high as 40 to 60 mg. per cent have been reported. As in the serum of the normal infant, the dominant pigment in erythroblastosis fetalis is unconjugated (indirect reacting) bilirubin, the presence of which in higher concentrations is capable of producing severe neurological damage, at least, during the first few days of life (*cf.* Kernicterus and Blood-brain barrier). (On the other hand, comparable quantities of conjugated [direct reacting] bilirubin appear to be better tolerated by the nervous system, as in congenital obliteration of the bile ducts and hepatitis of the newborn.) One of the aims of treatment by exchange transfusion is to control the degree of hyperbilirubinemia until the infant's enzymatic mechanisms for the conjugation of bilirubin have matured enough to halt the accumulation of unconjugated bilirubin in the blood serum.

Kernicterus; nuclear jaundice; bilirubin encephalopathy: Jaundice of the central nervous system, mainly of the basal nuclei of the brain, a common finding in erythroblastotic and in certain premature infants dying at the peak of their hyperbilirubinemia. There is a statistical correlation between the height of the bilirubin concentration and the occurrence of nuclear jaundice, so that when the bilirubin concentration is less than 20 mg. per cent the brain is rarely affected, but with bilirubin concentrations above 30 mg. per cent, as many as half such babies develop staining of the basal nuclei. Since brain damage is believed to be due to the toxic action of the indirect reacting bilirubin, it may occur also in babies who have little or no anemia. The incidence of kernicterus as a complication and cause of death in erythroblastosis fetalis can be markedly reduced by the judicious use of exchange transfusion, which temporarily lowers the concentration of bilirubin in the blood stream.

Neurologic sequelae: The most distressing sequel of erythroblastosis fetalis, occurring in babies with nuclear jaundice who survive. This may occur in as many as 5 to 10 per cent of babies, especially those not treated by exchange transfusion. Due to disseminated brain damage, such infants may exhibit severe mental and physical retardation, with athetosis and deafness as prominent signs.

Blood-brain barrier: The mechanism which normally prevents bilirubin and other substances from passing from the blood into the brain tissue and cerebro-spinal fluid. The barrier is believed to be less efficient at birth than it is in later life, and this accounts for the increased susceptibility of newborns to bilirubin encephalopathy. The mechanism matures with increasing age of the infant, but the precise time, if ever, when the danger of kernicterus associated with hyperbilirubinemia has passed is not known.

Inspissated bile syndrome: A rare complication of erythroblastosis fetalis characterized by acholic stools, bilirubinuria and a high concentration of direct-reacting bilirubin in the blood serum. Until recently, it was believed that in babies with hyperbilirubinemia large amounts of bile excreted by the liver occasionally became inspissated, producing blockage of the bile canaliculi. Observation of a pair of erythroblastotic male fraternal twins, only one of whom exhibited this syndrome, suggests that the predisposition is present at birth and is the result of the influence of certain as yet undefined constitutional factors. Affected babies usually recover, but frequently will have a green discoloration of the milk teeth when they erupt.

Hepatic necrosis: A rare, serious complication of erythroblastosis fetalis, which is responsible for the more intractable instances of hyperbilirubinemia. Most babies with this complication die, while the few that survive may later develop cirrhosis of the liver.

Antibodies in milk: Rh and other antibodies have been shown to be present in milk, especially in colostrum. Nevertheless, it is perfectly safe to permit erythroblastotic babies to nurse. After the first few days of life, the baby's stomach has the capacity to digest ingested milk proteins, so that only negligible amounts of undigested Rh antibodies are absorbed.

Exchange transfusion; exsanguination transfusion: A method of treatment of erythroblastosis, in which the affected baby's blood is withdrawn and simultaneously replaced by blood compatible with the maternal isoantibodies. The principal purpose of the operation is to remove the baby's coated red cells and replace them with red cells incapable of combining with the maternal antibodies present in the baby's body, and thus arresting the disease. When the procedure is promptly and correctly carried out, there is a significant reduction in the mortality rate and in the incidence of neurological sequelae among babies who survive. In addition to being more effective, exchange transfusion is more efficient than multiple small transfusions. The relationship between the volume of blood used for the exchange transfusion and the percentage exchange is given in table 18; the use of 2 pints of blood (four times the average newborn's blood volume) is recommended, resulting in a 98 per cent replacement. To increase the efficiency of the operation it is customary to begin by bleeding the baby of 30 to 60 cc., and this deficit is made up before the procedure is terminated. Post-transfusion anemia is avoided by removing part of the citrated plasma from the donor's blood in order to reduce the volume of each unit from 600 cc. (480 cc. of blood plus 120 cc. ACD solution) to about 450 cc. (hematocrit approximately 0.5). Blood used for exchange transfusion should not be more than 2 or 3 days old since blood stored for longer periods tends to accumulate dangerous potassium concentrations. The same volume of blood is transfused as is withdrawn, thus avoiding overloading or depleting the baby's circulation.

Indications for exchange transfusion: The decision whether or not to carry out exchange transfusion depends upon the serological findings together with the clinical manifestations. Babies who show

TABLE 18.—*Relationship Between Volume of Blood Used for Exchange Transfusion and the Percentage of Replacement of Blood**

Amount of Blood Exchanged in Units Equal to the Baby's Blood Volume	Percentage of Donor's Blood in Baby's Body after Transfusion
½ Blood volume..............................	39.4
1 Blood volume..............................	63.2
1½ Blood volumes.............................	77.7
2 Blood volumes.............................	86.5
2½ Blood volumes.............................	91.8
3 Blood volumes.............................	95.0
4 Blood volumes.............................	98.0

(Wiener, A. S., and Wexler, I. B.: J. Lab. & Clin. Med. *31:* 1016, 1946.)

* Formula: Percentage of donor's blood $= (1 - e^{-v}) \times 100$, where v is the amount of blood used for the exchange transfusion expressed in units equal to the baby's blood volume.

no anemia or jaundice are not treated even though the serological findings may be impressive. On the other hand, babies showing early deep jaundice should be exchanged even though the serological findings are mild. Hyperbilirubinemia is the chief indication for exchange transfusion, and some workers have even set a total serum bilirubin concentration of 20 mg. per cent as an absolute indication for treatment. However, there is nothing magical about this figure, and the decision whether or not to perform an exchange transfusion should rest not with the laboratory but with the clinician. Moreover, rather than wait until the bilirubinemia becomes extreme, an attempt should be made from the rate of rise of serum bilirubin concentration to determine whether or not a dangerous level is likely to be reached. Severe anemia at birth is an indication for exchange transfusion, though babies exhibiting severe anemia with little jaundice may also respond satisfactorily to simple transfusions of packed red blood cells.

Icterus index: A simple method of estimating the concentration of bilirubin in the blood serum. This is carried out by mixing a measured amount of the serum with an equal amount of acetone and removing the precipitated proteins by centrifugation. The supernatant is then diluted as necessary with distilled water and matched against artificial standards made with potassium dichromate. The icterus index is equal to the product of the matching standard and the dilution. Generally the icterus index is between five to seven times the bilirubin concentration in mg. per cent. The advantage of this test is its simplicity so that it may be carried out rapidly by the clinician himself, who is not at the mercy of the laboratory technician in making the decision whether or not to carry out the exchange transfusion, because it serves as a check on the accuracy of the bilirubin determination. Because of the close correlation between icterus index and total bilirubin, reliance can be placed on the icterus index alone. However, for maximum information, bilirubin determinations should also be done, especially to determine the proportions of direct- and indirect-reacting bilirubin.

Technic of exchange transfusion: Two main methods of exchange transfusion are in use, namely, the umbilical catheter method (Diamond), and the radial-artery/saphenous-vein method (Wiener and Wexler). In the former method, a translucent polyethylene catheter is passed through the umbilical vein into the inferior vena cava, and the baby's blood is removed and replaced by citrated type rh blood through the same catheter with the aid of a 10 or 20 cc. syringe. In the second method, type rh blood is injected by syringe into the saphenous vein at the ankle through a blunt 20 gauge needle, while the baby's blood is allowed to flow from a V-shaped incision made into the radial artery at the wrist. To facilitate bleeding, small doses of heparin are injected at the beginning of and during the transfusion, the effect of which has generally worn off by the time the procedure is completed. By either technic, 1 cc. of 10 per cent calcium gluconate is usually injected after every 100 cc. of blood transfused in order to counteract the effect of the citrate. The use of calcium makes it possible to carry out the procedure at a fairly rapid rate, namely, about 30 minutes for every unit of blood used.

The radial-artery/saphenous-vein technic has the advantage that it can be used on babies of any age; it is an open procedure and uses expendable vessels which are peripherally located, thus avoiding the dangers of hemoperitoneum, cardiac arrythmia and dilatation, air embolism, splenic rupture, and thrombosis of important vessels. The umbilical catheter method is the more widely used.

Suitable donors for erythroblastotic babies: Donors should belong to a compatible A-B-O blood group and lack the blood factor or factors present in the baby to which the mother is sensitized. Since, with rare exceptions, the only antibodies present in the newborn are those passively derived from the mother, the mother's red cells are always compatible, even when the baby belongs to group O and the mother to group A or group B. The mother's blood, or preferably the mother's washed red cells can therefore always be used for transfusions to their own newborn babies, and this is convenient when Rh-negative donors are not at hand, or in unusual cases such as those of **hr'** sensitization, or sensitization to more than one blood factor. For exchange transfusion for any case of erythroblastosis, the mother's cells suspended in compatible plasma is ideal. The mother may be bled into ACD solution, the plasma separated by centrifugation and reinjected into the mother, while the sedimented cells resuspended in plasma of group AB or of the mother's A-B-O group are used for the exchange transfusion. The father's blood is most unsuitable since it always contains the blood factor to which the mother is sensitized. Many workers routinely use low-titered group O, Rh-negative blood for all exchange transfusions to erythroblastotic babies. Rh-positive blood should never be used, even though it may be successful in mild cases. However, if the titer of free antibodies in the baby's serum is substantial, transfusions of Rh-positive blood will aggravate the disease. The sex of the donor appears to be inconsequential for the treatment of erythroblastotic babies.

Repeat exchange transfusion: The prime indication for repetition of the exchange transfusion is persistent hyperbilirubinemia. As has been pointed out (*cf.* Hyperbilirubinemia), the presence of excessive concentrations of indirect-reacting bilirubin in the blood stream can cause brain damage even in the absence of blood group incompatibility. By judicious timing and the use of a large volume of blood for each exchange transfusion, the number of exchange transfusions required can be minimized. Thus, the first transfusion is not necessarily given immediately after birth, but preferably 2 to 12 hours later depending upon the clinical condition of the infant and upon the rate of rise of the serum bilirubin concentration. Our own practice is to use two units of blood routinely (approximately 800–1,000 cc., or three to four blood volumes) except in mild cases where one unit may suffice. This generally reduces the serum bilirubin concentration to one-third or one-fourth of its original level. Within a few hours the bilirubin concentration rises (rebound phenomenon), due in large part to diffusion of bilirubin from the tissue spaces. If the bilirubin level continues to rise rapidly instead of reaching a plateau, a second exchange transfusion may be required. Two units are used again for this transfusion, and, on rare occasions, even three units. An attempt is made to withhold the second exchange transfusion for at least 24–36 hours after the first is completed. When these large volumes of blood are used with each exchange transfusion, the need for more than two procedures rarely arises.

Heparinized blood: Some workers have used heparinized blood, drawn immediately before the exchange transfusion, for the treatment of erythroblastotic babies. Other workers have added heparin to ACD blood and then treated it with enough calcium to neutralize the citrate, and used this for the transfusion. It is claimed that use of heparinized blood makes possible more rapid exchange transfusion, without the danger of cardiac arrest. Actually, the supposed advantages are only theoretical since bank blood less than 48–72 hours old coupled with the proper use of calcium gluconate gives as satisfactory results and avoids the problem of having to return a heparinized baby to the nursery.

Differential agglutination test: A test to determine the relative proportions of mixtures of bloods of different groups, used for tracing the survival of donor's cells in a recipient's circulation. It is also used to follow the course in an erythroblastotic baby following transfusion therapy. For example, if a group A recipient is transfused with group O cells, the patient's blood cells after the transfusion, mixed with anti-A serum, will exhibit clumps (the patient's cells) on a background of unagglutinated cells (the donor's cells), which can be counted in a blood counting chamber. Similarly, when the recipient and the donor belong to the same A-B-O blood group, but, for example, the donor belongs to type N and the recipient belongs to type MN, anti-**M** serum can be used to trace the donor's cells, etc. In performing these tests it is important to use antisera of high avidity which give a low inagglutinable cell count on normal blood.

Aregenerative phase: A period generally lasting 2 to 6 weeks after birth during which few new red cells are released from the bone marrow. This occurs in all newborn infants, but appears to be prolonged in erythroblastotic babies, probably due to the effect of the free Rh antibodies in the infant's plasma and body fluids which combine with the newly formed Rh-positive cells preventing their survival in the circulation, plus the bone-marrow supressive effect of the transfusions used in treatment. Thus, for the first few weeks after treatment by exchange transfusion, the red blood cell count and hemoglobin concentration fall while effete donor's cells are being eliminated. This rate of fall is exaggerated by the infant's increasing body size. During the aregenerative phase, the baby's blood types as Rh negative. Recovery is heralded by the appearance of reticulocytes in the blood smear, and Rh-positive cells in the differential agglutination test. The duration of the aregenerative phase appears to depend in part on the avidity and titer of the Rh antibodies in the baby's body, and if it is prolonged, a supplementary small transfusion of packed type rh cells may be necessary at about 4–6 weeks. For this transfusion a convenient donor is the mother, whose washed, packed, red blood cells may be routinely used. Hematinics for this phase have proved ineffectual.

hr' hemolytic disease: Erythroblastosis caused by maternal sensitization to the **hr'** factor. Sensitization to any of the known Rh-Hr factors can give rise to erythroblastosis fetalis, but aside from factor **Rh₀**, sensitization to factor **hr'** is responsible for more cases than all of the other Rh-Hr factors combined. Despite this, cases of **hr'** hemolytic disease are uncommon. Typically, the mother is type Rh₁Rh₁ and the child is type Rh₁rh (or rarely, type rh'rh). In these cases, the zygosity of the father with respect to the factor **hr'** can be determined serologically without the necessity of family studies. For example, individuals of type rh and Rh₀ are homozygous for factor **hr'**, while those of type Rh₁rh or RhzRh₀ are heterozygous. The principles of treatment are the same as those governing Rh-hemolytic disease, except that donors of type Rh₁Rh₁ are used for exchange transfusion instead of type rh donors.

Other causes of erythroblastosis fetalis: Sensitization to blood factors of blood group systems other than Rh-Hr have also given rise to hemolytic disease. The same principles of management are employed, and blood donors are selected who lack the factor in question.

When blood of an extremely rare type is needed for the exchange transfusion, maternal blood (*cf.* page 65) may be used for the first transfusion if needed to tide the infant over while other donors are being sought.

A-B-O hemolytic disease: The most common form of erythroblastosis fetalis aside from **Rh₀** hemolytic disease. In typical cases, the mother is group O and the baby is group A or group B. Unlike Rh-Hr hemolytic disease, the first born baby is frequently affected, and the direct antiglobulin (Coombs' test) is negative, or, at best, weakly positive. The blood film shows frequent spherocytes. In other respects (hyperbilirubinemia, anemia, hepatosplenomegaly, etc.) the clinical picture resembles that of Rh-Hr hemolytic disease (*cf.* table 19). However, since, in general, the manifestations are milder and spontaneous recovery is the rule, the need for exchange transfusion therapy occurs less commonly. As donors, group O individuals with low titer anti-**A** and anti-**B** isoantibodies are used. If time permits and facilities are available, washed group O red cells (or the mother's red cells) resuspended in plasma of group AB or of the baby's A-B-O blood group are ideal. Donors of the baby's own A-B-O blood group are to be avoided since the use of such blood aggravates the disease.

Serological varieties of A-B-O hemolytic disease: There appears to be two serological varieties of A-B-O hemolytic disease. In the more common variety, which affects the first born baby, the antibodies are the so-called natural isoantibodies which appear to be of the heterogenetic immune origin. These naturally occurring anti-**A** and anti-**B** isoagglutinins arise from the ingestion of foods or infection with microörganisms with A-like or B-like antigens. If the antibodies in the mother are of high enough titer and avidity, they may cause hemolytic disease in the baby. In the less common variety, the group O mother forms immune isoantibodies following a pregnancy with a group A or group B baby, so that subsequently born babies of an incompatible blood group may be affected. This variety, like Rh hemolytic disease, is generally more severe.

Secretors and non-secretors: A division of human beings into two hereditary types, depending on the presence or absence of blood group substances in the secretions and body fluids. For example, in group A individuals who are secretors, the blood group substance A

TABLE 19.—*Comparison of Rh-Hr and A-B-O Hemolytic Disease*

	Serologic Tests and Clinical Observations	Rh-Hr Hemolytic Disease	A-B-O Hemolytic Disease
Mother	A-B-O group	Any A-B-O blood group. Group O less frequent than in general population; group AB more frequent	Almost always group O
	Rh-Hr type	Nearly always **Rh**$_0$ neg. (**hr'** negative in **hr'** hemolytic disease)	May be any Rh-Hr type
	Serum antibodies	Serum contains **Rh**$_0$ antibodies (or **hr'**)	Serum has high titers of anti-**A** and/or anti-**B**, especially by acacia or antiglobulin technic
Father	A-B-O group	Compatible with mother's group more often than in other pregnancies	Always incompatible with mother's group
	Rh-Hr type	**Rh**$_0$ positive. (**hr'** positive in **hr'** hemolytic disease)	May be any Rh-Hr type
Baby	A-B-O group	Compatible with mother's group more often than in other pregnancies	Always incompatible with mother's A-B-O blood group
	Rh-Hr type	**Rh**$_0$ positive. (**hr'** positive in **hr'** hemolytic disease)	May be any Rh-Hr type
	Direct antiglobulin (Coombs') test.	Generally strongly positive	Generally negative or only weakly positive
	Order of birth	Generally 2nd or higher	Frequently occurs in first born child
	Severity of manifestations.	Generally severe	Generally mild
	Erythrocytes on blood smear	Macrocytic	Spherocytic

is demonstrated in high concentration in the saliva and other secretions, while in nonsecretors of group A, no blood group substance A is demonstrable. It has been suggested that most babies of group A or group B do not have A-B-O hemolytic disease when their mothers are group O because the babies are secretors, so that the maternal isoantibodies which reach their circulation are neutralized before they can combine with the baby's erythrocytes. Were this true, only nonsecretors would be affected. Actually it has been found that almost all babies who have A-B-O hemolytic disease are secretors, and there is evidence that the passage of the soluble antigen rather than the red cells is responsible for maternal hypersensitization, and that the secretor status of the infant has only limited protective effect. On the other hand, the incomplete development of the A-B-O agglutinogens on the red cells of the newborn does appear to be an important factor in the mildness of the manifestations in most cases of A-B-O hemolytic disease.

C sensitization: Sensitization to the blood factor **C** of the A-B-O blood group system. This appears to be the most common cause of A-B-O hemolytic disease as shown by the work of Rosenfield and of Wiener and Unger. The blood factor **C** has a position in the A-B-O system analogous to that of **Rh$_0$** in the Rh-Hr system. Thus, serum from group O individuals contains, in addition to anti-**A** and anti-**B**, a third agglutinin anti-**C** for a factor **C** shared by agglutinogens A and B. For reasons not as yet entirely clear, **C** antibodies appear to be capable of traversing the placental barrier more readily than **A** and **B** antibodies, and thus produce A-B-O hemolytic disease. This accounts for the observation that almost all mothers of babies affected with this disease belong to group O.

Prevention of erythroblastosis fetalis: No effective and universally satisfactory method of preventing erythroblastosis has been found to date. Artificial insemination with sperm from Rh-negative donors will, of course, prevent erythroblastosis caused by Rh sensitization, but suitable donors are difficult to obtain and the method suits the temperament of relatively few couples. Once the mother is sensitized, there is no known way of stopping the passage of the univalent antibodies through the placenta into the baby's circulation where they combine with the baby's red cells and bring about disease. As has been pointed out, in approximately one out of three normal pregnancies and deliveries, fetal blood enters the mother's circulation and brings about isosensitization, and no method of preventing this is known. Vitamin C, cortisone and ACTH have been tried without success. Some encouraging results were obtained by the use of counterimmunization (cf. Competition of antigens) but this method has not proved to be practicable. A substantial decrease in the incidence of erythroblastosis has taken place since the introduction of routine Rh typing when selecting blood for transfusion and the discontinuance of intramuscular injections of untyped blood. A further reduction has resulted from voluntary limiting the size of the family, when the mother is informed that she is isosensitized. Eugenic marriages between Rh-negative individuals are hardly the answer, since only one in twenty women become isosensitized, and there are more common causes of marital incompatibility than the Rh factor.

Competition of antigens: When an animal is injected with more than one antigen at the same time, the stronger antigen sometimes suppresses the immunizing effect of the weaker one. Wiener has suggested applying the principle to prevent erythroblastosis by counterimmunizing the expectant mother throughout pregnancy with potent but harmless vaccines such as typhoid and pertussis. The injections should be given regularly throughout the pregnancy, since proper timing is essential in order for competition of antigens to operate. The method is tedious and probably not suitable for general application, even though Unger and others have shown that it is effective in reducing the incidence of isosensitization. Obviously, the method is of no value for patients already sensitized, since in primed individuals Rh acts as a strong antigen (cf. Anamnestic reaction).

Hapten: A substance having the serological properties of antigens in in vitro tests, but without antigenic action in vivo (Landsteiner). Such haptens may be obtained, for example, by alcoholic extracts of organs. Alcoholic organ extracts when mixed with organ-specific antisera fix complement in vitro, but are nonantigenic for rabbits. When such organ extracts are mixed with carriers such as pig serum, they then become antigenic for rabbits.

Rh hapten: The specific nonantigenic portion of the Rh agglutinogen. It has been suggested that injection of Rh hapten into isosensitized pregnant Rh-negative mothers might protect the

Rh-positive fetus in utero. However, claims of the effectiveness of Rh hapten that have been published in the literature are invalid, since all preparations of so-called hapten obtained to date have proved to be devoid of specific activity both in vitro and in vivo. Had the original investigators used the blind test (*cf.* page 27), these claims would never have been published. Apparently, the Rh agglutinogen makes up only a very small portion of the red cell envelope, and attempts to extract it have so far been unsuccessful.

Infusion of Rh antiserum: The clinical value of passive immunization has proved practicable in measles, poliomyelitis, and certain bacterial infections. The injection of a large enough amount of antiserum on exposure to these diseases will not only temporarily prevent the disease, but also will not permit the development of active immunity. Similarly, it has been speculated that if an Rh-negative mother is given an intravenous injection of Rh antiserum immediately after delivery of an Rh-positive baby, this may prevent her from being sensitized to the Rh factor and thus avoid the occurrence of Rh hemolytic disease in future Rh-positive babies. This approach to the problem of the prophylaxis of hemolytic disease is still under investigation.

Postmortem diagnosis: In addition to kernicterus in erythroblastotic babies that die, jaundice, anemia, petechiasis, edema and hepatosplenomegaly are common findings, while histologic sections generally show numerous islands of hematopoiesis in the liver, spleen, and other organs. In stillbirths, the fetus may be shrunken and macerated and histologic examination is unsatisfactory; some stillborn fetuses are markedly enlarged due to hydrops and the placenta may be similarly enlarged. None of these findings is pathognomonic of erythroblastosis and the diagnosis can only be made reliably by typing the bloods of the father and the mother and demonstrating the presence of isosensitization by tests on the maternal serum.

Therapeutic abortion: This may be indicated in selected cases of Rh sensitization in pregnancy; for example, where in addition to a history of repeated erythroblastotic stillbirths, the expectant mother is strongly sensitized to the Rh factor, and the husband is homozygous Rh positive, making another stillbirth appear inevitable. Such pregnancies, besides being useless, carry an increased hazard to the mother, due to possible hydropic degeneration of the fetus with resulting toxemia. Moreover, the birth of such a fetus may be complicated by uncontrollable bleeding caused by leakage of tissue juices from the placental site into the maternal circulation, with resulting afibrinogenemia. When therapeutic abortion is carried out, sterilization should be done at the same time, if possible, to prevent the problem from arising again.

Medicolegal aspects of erythroblastosis fetalis: There are a number of medicolegal problems associated with the management of erythroblastosis fetalis. Needless to say, no physician can guarantee the results of therapy, but if a bad result can be ascribed to negligence, a suit for medical liability may result. In a number of cases substantial awards have been made to parents of babies with neurological sequelae, because of failure of the physician to carry out Rh typing on the mother, or suitable antibody tests on the Rh-negative expectant mother antenatally. Similarly, physicians in charge of the care of the infant have been sued for failure to carry out direct antiglobulin (Coombs') tests, bilirubin determinations and other pertinent tests on babies with neonatal jaundice for use as a guide to diagnosis and treatment. There have also been awards against hospitals for errors in typing which resulted in the transfusion of Rh-positive blood to Rh-negative women, thus bringing about sensitization.

CHAPTER V

Blood Transfusion

Intragroup hemolytic transfusion reactions: Hemolytic reactions occurring after transfusions of blood of the same A-B-O blood group as the recipient's. The most frequent cause of such reactions is the transfusion of Rh-positive blood to Rh-negative patients who have become sensitized to the **Rh₀** factor, as was first shown by Wiener and Peters. Therefore, it has become routine to include Rh testing in the pretransfusion tests, so that every Rh-negative recipient is given only Rh-negative blood, preferably type rh (*cf.* page 12). This precaution is essential not only to prevent hemolytic transfusion reactions but also to avoid sensitizing Rh-negative patients, especially women who may later give birth to an Rh-positive baby. In Rh-positive recipients, intragroup hemolytic reactions may be caused by sensitization to other Rh-Hr factors such as **hr′, rh′, rh″**, or blood factors of other blood group systems, notably **M, K**, and **F**.

Intragroup incompatibility: Incompatibility between individuals of the same A-B-O blood group; the cause of intragroup hemolytic reactions. The most common cause of intragroup incompatibility is isosensitization of Rh-negative recipients to the **Rh₀** factor, as can be detected by testing the patient's serum against standard Rh-positive cells. In Rh-positive recipients, intragroup incompatibility may be caused by sensitization to other blood factors such as **hr′, rh′, rh″, M, S, K**, and **F**. Intragroup incompatibility caused by sensitization to more than one blood factor, e.g., **Rh₀** and **M, Rh₀** and **K**, etc. may also be encountered; therefore, it is advisable to keep on hand a panel of donors who have been fully classified for the more important blood group systems, in order to resolve such difficult transfusion problems. A summary of the known blood group systems and blood factors which have been shown to exist up to the present time is given in table 20.

TABLE 20.—*Blood Factors of Human Blood Known in 1962*

Blood Group Systems	Blood Factors
1. A-B-O	A, A_1, B_i, B_{ii}, B_{iii}, ..., H, C, F_A, A^P, ...
2. Lewis	Le^a, Le^b, Le^x, Le^c, ...
3. M-N-S	M_i, M_{ii}, M_{iii}, M_{iv}, ..., N_i, N_{ii}, ..., S, s, U, Hu, He, M^e, Gr, Mi^a, Mu, ..., M^g, M_1, Vr, Mt^a, Ri^a, St^a, ...
4. Rh-Hr	Rh_0, Rh^A, Rh^B, Rh^C, Rh^D, ..., rh', rh^{w_1}, rh^x, rh^G, ..., rh'', rh^{w_2}, rh^T, ..., hr', hr'', hr^S, ..., hr, rh_i, rh, ..., Hr, hr^V, hr^N, ...
5. P	P, Tj^a, P^k, ...
6. Kell	K, k, Kp^a, Kp^b, Ku, ...
7. Duffy	Fy^a, Fy^b, ...
8. Kidd	Jk^a, Jk^b, ...
9. Lutheran	Lu^a, Lu^b, ...
10. Diego	Di^a, ...
11. Sutter	Js^a, Js^b, ...
12. I	I, i, ...
13. Auberger	Au^a, ...
14. Sex-linked	Xg^a, ...
15. Others:	
High frequency factors:	Vel, Yt^a, Ge, Ge^Y, Lan, Sm, Pearl, Cartw., Bout., Ters., ...
Low frequency factors:	Ca, Be^a, Becker, Ven, Rm, By, Levay, Sw^a, Good, Bi, Tr^a, Wb, Chr^a, Stobo, Ot, Ho, Price, ...

Number of human blood groups: If every one of the 103 blood factors listed in table 20 were independent of one another, they would give rise to 2^{103} or 10^{31} blood types. This, of course, would be far more than enough to fulfill Landsteiner's prediction of the complete individuality of human blood, since this would imply the existence of more than a sextillion blood types for every living person. Obviously, if blood had to be matched with regard to all known blood factors, blood transfusion would be impossible.

In practice, however, the extent to which a person's blood can be individualized is disappointing. Firstly, hardly any laboratory has more than 20 of the reagents listed in the table. Secondly, certain blood factors are almost universal in their distribution, e.g., **I**, **Vel**, **U**,

Tj^a, etc., while others are very rare. The most important phenomenon limiting the number of different blood types is the inheritance of certain blood factors in blocks, e.g., blood has either all or none of the factors **B**$_i$, **B**$_{ii}$, **B**$_{iii}$, etc. Similarly, all M blood has the factors **M**$_i$, **M**$_{ii}$, **M**$_{iii}$, etc., while *almost* all Rh-positive blood has all of the associated factors **Rh**^{A}, **Rh**^{B}, **Rh**^{C}, etc.

Naturally occurring isoantibodies: Isoantibodies in general may be divided into two main categories; namely, those which occur spontaneously and those which result from immunization by transfusions or pregnancy. The most important naturally occurring isoantibodies are anti-**A** and anti-**B** whose regular presence in individuals lacking the corresponding agglutinogen makes A-B-O grouping an essential preliminary to blood transfusion. Other isoantibodies which may occur spontaneously, but much less frequently, are anti-**H**, anti-**Le**, anti-**M**, anti-**N** and anti-**P**. In general, spontaneously occurring antibodies react more strongly at low temperatures. They appear to be of heterogenetic immune origin.

Isoimmune antibodies: Antibodies which result from immunization by blood transfusion or other blood injection, or by pregnancy. Such antibodies generally react best at body temperature and may be demonstrated by a variety of technics, notably, the antiglobulin method. Of these antibodies, the most important are those determining the blood factors of the Rh-Hr system. Less frequently, incompatibility and hemolytic transfusion reactions may be caused by members of the Kell, Duffy, Kidd, M-N-S, and P systems.

Pretransfusion blood grouping: Obviously it would be impracticable to type patients for all blood factors which can give rise to isosensitization and hemolytic transfusion reactions, and, fortunately, this is not necessary. It is generally sufficient to classify patients for the four A-B-O groups and for the blood factor **Rh**$_0$ (making a total of eight blood types), and to select a donor of the corresponding type. To prevent reactions caused by other blood factors, reliance is placed on crossmatching tests. Even the limited division of patients and donors into only eight blood types causes difficulties because of the unequal distribution of the blood types. The most difficult of the eight types of blood to obtain, of course, is group AB, Rh negative, which has an incidence of less than 1 per cent.

Crossmatching tests: Tests in which the plasma (or serum) of the recipient is mixed with the red cells of the prospective donor, and the plasma (or serum) of the prospective donor is mixed with the red cells of the recipient; after incubation, the mixtures are examined for the presence or absence of clumping. The purpose of this test is to detect intragroup incompatibility; at the same time the test serves as a further check on the accuracy of the A-B-O and Rh typings. If no clumping occurs in either mixture, the donor is compatible and his blood may be used for the transfusion.

The mixture containing the patient's serum and donor's cells is called the major match (or major side of the crossmatch), while the other mixture is called the minor match. The major match is far more important because the introduction of incompatible cells rather than of incompatible plasma is the usual cause of hemolytic reactions. Incompatible plasma is rapidly diluted by the recipient's own plasma, while incompatible cells bear the full brunt of the hemolytic action of the recipient's plasma. In fact, in some blood banks only matching of the recipient's plasma with the donor's cells is carried out.

If the patient has been isosensitized, the isoantibodies will be more often of the univalent than the bivalent form; therefore, in addition to the matching tests by the agglutination method on saline-suspended cells, methods of matching designed to detect univalent antibodies must also be carried out. Of these, the most convenient is the conglutination (*cf.* p. 18) crossmatch, carried out, for example, as follows: An applicator is inserted into a clot of the donor's blood and then transferred to a small tube containing one or two drops of the recipient's serum; in this way enough donor's cells are transferred to make a 2 to 5 per cent suspension in patient's serum. A drop of 30 per cent bovine albumin is added, and the mixture allowed to stand for 5 to 10 minutes, preferably at body temperature. The tube is then centrifuged at low speed for 1 minute, the tube shaken to dislodge the sediment, and then examined for clumping. Treatment of the prospective donor's cells by proteolytic enzymes (*cf.* p. 25) is ideal for detecting Rh-Hr incompatibility but is perhaps too laborious for routine use; besides, the enzymes damage the M-N agglutinogens so that the test is not suitable for detecting isosensitization to them. The most sensitive method of matching is the antiglobulin (Coombs') technic (*cf.* page 23) which also detects the rare isoantibodies anti-**K**, anti-**F** (anti-**Duffy**) and anti-**J** (anti-**Kidd**) which are not detected as readily by the conglutination test. The antiglobulin method must be used to determine the nature of the incompatibility whenever intragroup hemolytic transfusion reactions occur.

Diagnosis of intragroup hemolysis: Clinically, this should be suspected whenever a recently transfused patient has any or all of the following symptoms: chill, fever, shock, hemoglobinuria, hemoglobinemia, jaundice, anuria, oliguria, and azotemia. If the patient and the donor belong to different M-N types, the rapid elimination of the donor's cells from the patient's circulation can be demonstrated by differential agglutination tests. The diagnosis is established by demonstrating the presence in the recipient's serum of an antibody which clumps the donor's cells but not the recipient's own cells. To establish the specificity of the isoantibody in the patient's serum, as complete typing as possible should be carried out, in order to determine what blood factors are present in the donor's cells which are absent from the patient's cells. For example, if the recipient belongs to type O N.S Rh_1rh pp kk ff and the donor to type O M.S Rh_2rh P K F, one must consider the possibility of sensitization to blood factors **rh″**, **M**, **K**, **F**, and **P**. The specificity of the antibody or antibodies in the recipient's serum is then determined by testing the serum against a panel of blood specimens, some containing and others lacking the blood factors in question. If facilities are not available for such a detailed analysis, one of the central blood grouping laboratories, or a worker in the field should be consulted. Such problems are important research material, and indeed it is by the study of such cases that new blood factors have been discovered in the past. Luckily, most recipients do not become isosensitized to the blood factors lacking from their bloods even if they are repeatedly transfused with blood which contains the factors. The capacity to react to the infusion of incompatible blood appears to be governed by constitutional factors as yet to be defined, so that while some persons develop no sensitization at all, others become sensitized to multiple factors more often than can be attributed to chance alone (*cf.* multiple sensitization).

Multiple sensitization: Sensitization to more than one blood factor at a time. Aside from certain common double sensitizations such as Rh_0 and **M**, Rh_0 and **K**, **rh′** and **hr″**, and **rh″** and **hr′**, it has been observed that multiple sensitization to poorly antigenic blood factors occurs more frequently than can be attributed to chance alone. Such observations indicate the existence of individuals with an inordinate ability to become isoimmunized (and autoimmunized), notably patients with acquired hemolytic anemia, in lupus erythematosus, in lymphomata, and in cirrhosis of the liver. Instances have been reported in which recipients of multiple transfusions have become isosensitized to as many as five or more poorly antigenic blood factors. In fact, it has been by the study of such patients that several new blood factors have been discovered (Callender and Race).

Selection of donors for isosensitized patients: Once one has established the identity of the antibody responsible for a transfusion reaction and the incompatibility in the crossmatch tests, it becomes possible to select appropriate compatible donors for further transfusions, if needed. For example, patients sensitized to the **hr'** factor may be given type Rh_1Rh_1 blood; those sensitized to factor **M** are given type N blood, etc. Certain types of sensitization pose serious problems because of the extremely low frequency of compatible donors; for example, a patient sensitized to factor **k** requires type $\underline{K}K$ blood which has a frequency of only 1 in 500. Persons of type $\underset{=}{Rh_0}$ or $\underset{=}{Rh^w}$ require blood of the corresponding type which is even rarer, while sensitized **Vel**-negative patients depend upon donors having an incidence of about 1 in 5,000. Other rare examples are those persons of type rh'rh' who have become doubly sensitized to blood factors Rh_0 and **hr'**.

It may be possible by testing siblings or other close relatives of the patient to find others of the patient's type. Otherwise, recourse must be had to the central file of rare donors of the American Association of Blood Banks or to some other similar agency for information regarding donors of the desired type.

Treatment of hemolytic transfusion reactions: No treatment is required in most cases, since, contrary to the common conception, hemolysis of the transfused incompatible blood is often gradual and the products of hemolysis are readily disposed of. Even when acute hemolysis occurs, transfusions of less than 150 cc. of incompatible blood are generally not dangerous. Nevertheless, one or two 50 cc. ampoules of sodium citrate should be injected intravenously in order to alkalinize the urine and thus reduce the likelihood of hemoglobinuric nephrosis. On the other hand, large transfusions of incompatible blood are always serious, so that if the patient is seen early, energetic treatment in the form of exchange transfusions to remove as much of the incompatible blood as possible should be considered. Unfortunately, the carrying out of such a procedure is not always possible because of the large amount of compatible blood required for exchange transfusion in an adult. After anuria sets in it is a common mistake to treat the patient with large amounts of intravenous fluids with the expectation that the resulting hypervolemia will start a diuresis. Actually, such treatment aggravates the already present derangement of fluid and electrolyte balance, and hastens death from cerebral edema. Best results are obtained by limiting fluids to about 1,000 cc. a day, and maintaining the patient in the best electrolyte balance possible under the circumstances. If facilities are available, placing the patient on an artificial kidney may tide him over until renal function returns. In general, the prognosis in hemolytic transfusion reactions depends mainly on the quantity of incompatible blood transfused, and the potency of the isoantibodies in the recipient's plasma. The mortality rate in cases of anuria may be as high as 50 per cent, but this can be considerably reduced by rational treatment.

Postmortem diagnosis of hemolytic transfusion reactions: This generally depends upon the demonstration of a hemoglobinuric nephrosis; liver necrosis is another not uncommon finding. While hemoglobinuric nephrosis is generally considered pathognomonic of transfusion hemolysis, it may be encountered in other conditions, notably the so-called crush syndrome. In view of the medico-legal implications of transfusion hemolysis, the pathologist should weigh the evidence carefully before offering such a diagnosis, unless there is serological evidence of incompatibility to support his impression.

Emergency transfusion: In the emergencies arising after acute hemorrhage, there may not be sufficient time to perform all the grouping and crossmatching tests essential to make transfusion safe. In such contingencies, "universal donor" blood, namely, group O, Rh-negative blood is often used in order to save the time required to type and cross-match the blood of the recipient. If Rh-negative blood is not available, Rh-positive group O blood is sometimes used, but only if tests prove that the recipient is not sensitized to the Rh factor. Under these circumstances, the dangers of inducing Rh sensitization should be weighed against the danger of death from bleeding, and if the decision is made to proceed with the transfusion under these emergency conditions, a note should be entered on the chart to justify and explain the course of action taken. Since group O blood with a high titer of isoagglutinins may be dangerous for recipients not belonging to group O, Witebsky has advised adding soluble A and B group substances to neutralize the isoagglutinins. However, it has been found that the group substances do not neutralize the isoagglutinins sufficiently when the titer is very high, and besides group substances may isosensitize female group O recipients to the A and B agglutinogens and complicate subsequent pregnancies. It is safer to titrate the isoagglutinins and set aside group O blood of low titer for use as "safe universal donor blood," or, better, to remove the plasma and replace it with group AB plasma. Pooled plasma is often used to tide the patient over in emergencies until compatible blood becomes available, but pooled plasma not infrequently causes homologous serum jaundice and can also sensitize recipients to the A and B agglutinogens. Therefore, the use of "plasma expanders" such as dextran has been advocated for use in emergencies, but this also has disadvantages. Whatever course the transfusionist adopts during an emergency, he should type the blood of the recipient while the emergency infusion is running, so that compatible blood can be made available as quickly as possible in the event that further treatment will be required.

Homologous serum hepatitis: A variety of hepatitis resulting from transfusion of whole blood or plasma or of other material containing human serum. It is believed to be due to the transmission of a virus from the apparently healthy donor to the recipient, and is recognized by its characteristic incubation period of 60 to 120 days following the injection. The virus has not yet been isolated and cannot be transmitted to animals. Unfortunately, there is no reliable diagnostic test whereby healthy carriers of the virus can be identified, and no known processing of whole blood which will reliably destroy the virus without damaging the blood. Freezing and drying of plasma preserves the virus, while pooling increases the chances of transmission. Evidence has been adduced that keeping pooled plasma at room temperature for 6 months or longer inactivates the virus and renders such plasma safe for transfusion. During World War II, transfusion of pooled plasma was followed by the occurrence of hepatitis in as many as 10 per cent of cases, and the incidence of this complication has been reported to be from 1 in 500 to 1 in 50 following transfusion of whole blood. Since homologous serum hepatitis may be fatal, this complication may have medicolegal implications. However, no award has ever been made by a court in such a medicolegal case, since the complication is considered to be a calculated risk of blood transfusion.

Indications for transfusion: The main indication for blood transfusion is to replace blood loss following trauma, surgery and delivery. The use of blood transfusion for its "general tonic" effect or for such medical indications as secondary anemia is to be condemned. The only exceptions are certain blood dyscrasias such as leukemia, aplastic anemia, refractory anemia, Cooley's anemia, and hemophilia, where transfusions may help to prolong life. Transfusion must not be considered a minor procedure because of the occasional development of hemolytic reactions and the transmission of homologous serum hepatitis. In fact, where an unnecessary transfusion has caused the death of a patient as the result of an error in blood grouping, the courts have held the physician who ordered the procedure equally responsible with the blood bank and the hospital. Some surgeons refuse to operate unless the patient's hemoglobin concentration has a certain minimal value. This practice has resulted in wide variations in the number of transfusions given at different hospitals, due to differences in the methods of determining hemoglobin concentrations. This is only one example of the lack of discrimination in selecting patients who require blood transfusion.

Non-hemolytic transfusion reactions: Reactions to transfusion which cannot be accounted for by red blood cell incompatibility. Some of the reactions appear to be allergic in nature, and are characterized by urticaria in the milder cases, by wheezing in the more severe cases, and in some extremely rare instances by anaphylactic shock. Such reactions are thought to be due to sensitivity of the recipient to some allergen present in the donor's serum, as following food ingestion, and are treated by injections of small amounts of adrenalin. Chills and fever in the absence of blood group incompatibility have been traced to pyrogens present in the solutions and apparatus used in the processing and administration of the blood, but such pyrogenic reactions have been virtually eliminated by the use of modern expendable transfusion apparatus. According to some workers, many of these reactions are due to isosensitization of the patient to platelets and leukocytes. However, the reported attempts to demonstrate such platelet and leukocyte antibodies are unconvincing, because of the tendency of suspensions of platelets and leukocytes to undergo spontaneous clumping. At any rate, the tests are poorly reproducible, and the proponents of this point of view admit that there is little or no correlation between the results of the tests and the occurrence of transfusion reactions. In patients who are prone to pyrogenic reactions, the administration of 5 to 10 gr. of aspirin may prevent the reaction. This should be given at the onset of the infusion, which should not be prolonged beyond 60 to 90 minutes. If this fails, transfusion of packed or, better, of suitably prepared washed red cells may avoid a reaction by eliminating all substances other than red cells.

CHAPTER VI

Autosensitization and Acquired Hemolytic Anemia

Immunologic tolerance: Immunologic paralysis, or the inability to react immunologically to specific antigenic material growing within or present in large amounts in the body. This phenomenon is actually related to the principle of *"horror autotoxicus"* enunciated by Paul Ehrlich at the turn of the century—that is, the inability of the body to form antibodies against its own constituents. Exceptions to this were soon found, notably, the ability to sensitize to lens protein either experimentally or clinically, as in cases of sympathetic ophthalmia, although such sensitization was explained away as being caused by antigens that were outside of the body proper. Felton later showed that mice injected with massive amounts of type III pneumococcus polysaccharide could no longer react to type III polysaccharide, so that infections with small doses of type III pneumococcus proved to be fatal. Such mice could still react against pneumococci of other types. This highly specific inability to react to antigens Felton called immunologic paralysis. Owen in his observations on blood group mosaics in cattle twins introduced the term immunologic tolerance. It would appear that *"horror autotoxicus,"* immunologic paralysis, and immunologic tolerance are all different aspects of the same phenomenon, a characteristic of which is that tolerance exists only as long as significant amounts of the specific antigen remain in the body. This has been demonstrated, for example, in experiments with massive injections of soluble antigens in newborn animals.

Autosensitization; autoimmunization: The state of being immunized or sensitized to some constituent of the individual's own body. Contrary to the opinion formerly held, it is possible under certain conditions for antibodies to be formed against constituents of an individual's own body. These instances manifestly represent a failure of immunologic tolerance. The prefix *"auto"* is to a certain extent a misnomer, since such antibodies generally react with antigens shared by *every* member of the species, so that the antibodies are actually species specific and are not merely autoantibodies. Autosensitization is the cause of certain previously obscure clinical states, such as acquired hemolytic anemia (autoantibodies for red cells), certain types of nephritis (autoantibodies for kidney), Hoshimoto's disease (autoantibodies for thyroid), encephalitis (autoantibodies for brain), and idiopathic thrombocytopenic purpura (autoantibodies for platelets). They may also play a part in pemphigus (autoantibodies for skin) and disseminated lupus erythematosus. In lupus, antibodies have been demonstrated for DNA as well as for red blood cells.

Acquired autohemolytic anemia: An anemia occurring at any age which can be traced to the formation of autoantibodies for red blood cells. These have been divided into two main categories, depending on whether the autoantibodies react at body temperature (warm autoantibodies) or at refrigerator temperature (cold autoantibodies). In most cases the disease seems to develop spontaneously for no known antecedent cause. It is then termed idiopathic acquired hemolytic anemia. Occasionally it arises as a complication of another disease, notably virus or atypical pneumonia. Of the two serological forms, the one associated with warm autoantibodies is the more common.

Warm autoantibodies: A variety of autoantibody reacting with equal or greater intensity and titer at body than at refrigerator temperature. Such antibodies do not occur normally, but appear to be produced only by certain individuals who have a remarkable capacity to produce antibodies. Because the antibodies react at body temperature, they are capable of destroying the individual's own red cells in vivo, and may give rise to a disease which in certain important respects resembles erythroblastosis fetalis. The warm autoantibodies, like Rh antibodies, occur in both the univalent and bivalent forms, the univalent being by far the more common. They are 7S globulins, which coat the patient's own red cells, giving rise to a positive direct antiglobulin reaction, as in Rh-Hr hemolytic disease. In addition, autoantibodies in many instances can be demonstrated free in the serum, using the same technics as for Rh-Hr antibodies, notably the conglutination, antiglobulin, and enzyme-treated cell technics.

Because red cells which have been maximally coated with warm autoantibodies react with antiglobulin serum to the same titer as cells maximally coated with Rh-Hr antibodies, A. S. Wiener has suggested that warm autoantibodies react with that portion of the Rh-Hr molecule which is common to all Rh-Hr types. However, W. Weiner has shown that occasionally autoantibodies may be specific for a blood factor present in the individual's own red cells. As is to be expected, therefore, such type specific autoantibodies are most often of specificity anti-**hr**″, though autoantibodies of other specificities, notably anti-**rh**′, alone, or in combination, have also been described. Not infrequently, when tests are carried out with nonspecific warm autoantibodies using enzyme-treated red cells, lysis instead of agglutination occurs. If the serum is inactivated by heating at 56 C. for one-half hour, or by aging, it loses its ability to lyse cells, but continues to clump them. Autoantibodies of still other specificities may conceivably exist; for example, there is evidence supporting the existence of rare autoantibodies which react with the nucleus of the M-N substance—that is, the portion of the M-N agglutinogens which individuals of all M-N types have in common.

Normal cold autoantibodies: These are autoantibodies present in the serum of virtually every normal human being. Except during the first months of life, almost everyone has autoantibodies in his serum capable of clumping his own red cells. These autoantibodies are of low titer and avidity and react only at low temperature; in many instances they are demonstrable only when enzyme-treated cells are used. Circumstantial evidence suggests that the natural cold autoantibodies, as well as the A-B-O blood group isoantibodies, are of heterogenetic immune origin, and are due to inapparent infections with microörganisms having polysaccharides similar to the blood group mucopolysaccharides. This is supported by the rise in cold autoantibody titer in certain specific infections, notably atypical pneumonia (for which cold autoantibody titer is used as a diagnostic test), leishmaniasis, trypanosomiasis, tropical eosinophilia, and mumps. Wiener and Mollison both believe that the cold autoantibodies react with the A-B-O blood group mucopolysaccharides, but are specific for that portion of the molecule which individuals of all blood groups have in common. This idea is supported by the observation that associated with the cold autoantibodies, cold antibodies of specificities anti-A_1, anti-H, and anti-Le[a] are not infrequently present.

Abnormal cold autoantibodies: Cold autoantibodies of extraordinarily high titer, such as are found in association with acquired hemolytic anemia. Some of the highest titers of red cell antibodies are found when titrating these autoantibodies at refrigerator temperature, yet the antibodies react with only moderate titers at room temperature, and not at all, or only weakly, at body temperature. The titers in some cases have reached as high as 500,000 units, and in such cases a large abnormal peak can be demonstrated on electrophoresis, proving the presence of significant quantities of an abnormal serum globulin, distinct from normal gamma globulin. By ultracentrifugation these antibodies have been characterized as 19S macroglobulins. Cold autoantibodies, like warm autoantibodies, generally occur for no evident cause in so-called idiopathic acquired hemolytic anemia and/or Raynaud's syndrome, but also not infrequently in lymphomatous conditions such as lymphosarcoma and lymphatic leukemia. In some cases of autohemolytic anemia, associated with the potent cold autoantibodies there have been found type specific antibodies for a blood factor I of almost universal distribution.

Acquired hemolytic anemia: An anemia caused by a hemolytic agent, as distinguished from the purely hereditary hemolytic anemias. Acquired hemolytic anemia may result from the ingestion of certain drugs and plant products by persons with glucose-6-phosphate dehydrogenase deficiency, or from infection with microörganisms which produce hemolysins, or it may occur without apparent cause. In many cases of idiopathic acquired hemolytic anemia it has been possible to demonstrate the presence of an abnormal antibody in the patient's serum which coats the red cells.

Just as there are two forms of autoantibodies, warm and cold, so there are two major varieties of autohemolytic anemia. The acquired hemolytic anemia characterized by the presence of warm autoantibodies serologically resembles erythroblastosis fetalis, except that the antibodies in acquired hemolytic anemia are actively produced by the patient's own body, instead of being passively acquired as they are in erythroblastosis. The diagnosis, as in Rh-Hr hemolytic anemia, is made by the direct antiglobulin (Coombs') test, and by demonstrating the presence of the abnormal antibodies in the patient's serum. However, since the patient is actively sensitized he may continue to produce the antibodies indefinitely, while the erythroblastotic infant's disease is in this sense at least self-limiting, with the passively acquired antibodies being eliminated over a period of a few weeks or months. Autohemolytic anemia caused by cold autoantibodies may also persist for an indefinite period of time. The characteristic feature here, however, is the sensitivity to cold and the associated vascular phenomena. On exposure to cold, intravascular clumping may occlude the smaller blood vessels, producing the so-called Raynaud's syndrome, which may progress to gangrene of the tips of the fingers, toes and lobes of the ears if the exposed parts are not warmed promptly. Hematologically, the patient may present initially in an acute hemolytic crisis with severe anemia and even hemoglobinuria. On recovery from the acute attack, the blood may continue to show an anemia, hyperbilirubinemia and high reticulocytosis for a period of many years.

Pathogenesis prevention and treatment of acquired hemolytic anemia due to warm autoantibodies: Why autoantibodies are formed is unknown, and no method is known of preventing the disease. A constitutional predisposition appears to be present, as shown by the higher incidence of females than males among affected individuals. As has been pointed out, once autoimmunization has occurred, the production of autoantibodies generally continues indefinitely, and no method of treatment is known which can affect this. Accordingly, the disease is a chronic one, characterized by remissions and relapses, and complete recovery is exceptional. During the acute hemolytic phase or crisis, blood transfusion may be lifesaving, but repeated transfusions may be required before remission occurs. However, transfusion is a double-edged sword, since the autoantibodies in the patient's plasma may hemolyze the donor's cells so that transfusions often aggravate instead of helping the situation. The selection of donors compatible in in vitro tests is always difficult and often impossible; paradoxically, donors of Rh-Hr types opposite to that of the patient may prove most suitable. For example, in cases where the autoantibodies exhibit type specificity such as anti-**hr''**, donors of types Rh_2Rh_2 should be used, but this type has an incidence of only about 2 per cent so that such donors are difficult to obtain. In desperate cases the only recourse may be to use the blood which gives the weakest reactions with the patient's serum, and to premedicate the patient with antipyretics.

Steroid therapy appears to ameliorate the hemolytic process, even though it has no obvious effect on the production of the autoantibodies. Exchange transfusion, which theoretically would remove some of the autoantibodies as well as the susceptible recipient red blood cells, has been tried, but the results have been disappointing. In desperate cases, splenectomy has also been tried, either with no beneficial effect, or at most only temporary remission of the hemolytic process. It is interesting that some patients have prolonged remissions with entirely normal hematologic findings despite the presence of serological evidence of potent autosensitization. This indicates that some factor or factors in addition to the autoantibodies play an important role in this disease.

Pathogenesis and treatment of autohemolytic anemia due to cold autoantibodies: As with warm autoantibody disease, the pathogenesis of hemolytic anemia due to cold autoantibodies is generally unknown, except perhaps in cases which are associated with atypical pneumonia and infectious mononucleosis. The presence of cold autoantibodies in these cases suggests that the antibodies may be of heterogenetic immune origin. The acquired hemolytic anemia associated with atypical pneumonia tends to be benign and self-limited, and as a rule no transfusion therapy is required. The idiopathic type, in which there is an association with one of the lymphomata, is more grave and may run a rapid course with a high mortality rate. Transfusion may be helpful during hemolytic crises, but steroid therapy and splenectomy have not proved to be beneficial. The patient must avoid exposure to cold, and it may be necessary for him to move to a warm climate.

Disseminated lupus erythematosus: An obscure chronic disease occurring predominantly in females, characterized by bouts of fever, arthritic manifestations, skin lesions—especially a butterfly rash on the cheeks and nose—hemolytic anemia, thrombocytopenic purpura, jaundice, atypical verrucose endocarditis (Libman-Sacks), nephritis, and cerebral manifestations. Affected individuals generally have a persistently elevated sedimentation rate, and an inversion in the albumin-globulin ratio of the serum. Disseminated lupus erythematosus is believed to be due to widespread organ autosensitization, with red blood cell autosensitization and hemolytic anemia as only one aspect of the process. As to be expected, in certain cases the direct antiglobulin reaction is positive; however, the degree of coating is usually mild. The L. E. cell phenomenon (Hargraves) has been attributed to the reaction of autoantibodies with DNA. Thrombotic thrombocytopenic purpura appears to be another manifestation of the action of the autoantibodies in this disease.

CHAPTER VII
Anthropologic Aspects

Classification of human populations: While no single Rh-Hr type appears to be restricted to, or is characteristic of any ethnic group, the distribution of the Rh-Hr types is not the same in human populations in different parts of the world (*cf.* table 4). The situation is similar to that observed previously for the A-B-O groups and M-N types, except that the differences are far more striking in the case of the Rh-Hr types. Based on these differences in the distribution of the blood group factors, Wiener has suggested a semiqualitative classification of human races as is shown in table 21.

Rh gene frequencies: The percentage frequencies of the Rh genes in a population. These can be calculated from the frequencies of the phenotypes with the aid of the formulae given on page 33. As can be seen, tests with the three Rh antisera, anti-Rh_0, anti-rh', and anti-rh'' alone, give enough information to permit calculation of the gene frequencies. Tests with the Hr antisera are not essential, but are useful for confirming the calculations. When comparing populations, gene frequencies are more informative than phenotype frequencies. In table 22 are given the Rh gene frequencies for a number of representative human populations throughout the world. The striking differences among the three main racial subdivisions of mankind are apparent. Caucasians are characterized by the highest frequency of gene r, Negroes by the very high frequency of gene R^0, while in Mongolians gene r tends to be absent and the rare gene R^z has its highest frequency. These findings confirm the view that Amerindians and Australian aborigenes are of Mongolian origin. Moreover, they indicate that Papuans probably do not owe their dark skin color to African components, but belong to the Mongolian division of mankind.

Selection against heterozygotes: Isosensitization by pregnancy and the resulting death of erythroblastotic babies has a selective

TABLE 21.—*Classification of Human Races, Based on the Distribution of the Blood Group Factors (Wiener)*

I. Caucasoid group
   Highest frequency of gene r
   A_2 present as well as A_1
   Gene M slightly more frequent than gene N

II. Negroid group
   Highest frequency of gene R^0, also highest frequency of factor $\Re h_0$
   A_2 present as well as A_1; also frequent intermediates ($A_{1,2}$)
   Gene M and gene N about equally frequent

III. Mongoloid group—Highest frequency of rare gene R^Z and lowest frequency of gene r
   A_2 absent
   a) Asiatic subdivision—Genes M and N about equal
   b) Pacific subdivision (including Australian aborigines and Ainu)—low frequency of gene M, high frequency of gene N
   c) American subdivision (including Amerindians and Eskimos)— high frequency of gene M, low frequency of gene N

action against babies heterozygous for the **Rh**$_0$ factor, e.g., genotypes R^1r and R^2r. Thus, an equal number of Rh-positive genes (Rh) and Rh-negative genes (rh) are lost by the human race every generation. If, initially, the genes Rh and rh are equal in frequency, this selective process will not disturb their relative proportions. But, as Wiener and Haldane have pointed out, if their frequencies are unequal, the process has a relatively greater effect on the less frequent gene, so that after thousands of generations the less frequent gene would tend to be eliminated. In view of these considerations it becomes necessary to explain the frequency of 40 per cent for gene rh among Caucasians. Wiener has suggested that this unstable high frequency was the result of crossing some time in the past between two or more populations, one with a low frequency of gene rh (such as the Mongolians) and the other with a high frequency of gene rh (hypothetic proto-Europeans). This hypothesis has received some support from the findings on Basques, who have the highest frequency of gene rh (up to 60 per cent and higher) observed to date. Thus the modern Basques, isolated from invasion in the past by the Pyrenees, appear to represent the last vestiges of the hypothetic proto-Europeans. Similar populations have been found in Alpine villages.

Racial crossing: If a hybrid population is the result of a cross between two or more populations, and the Rh gene frequencies of the parent populations are known, as well as the proportions of the parent populations which took part in the cross, then the Rh gene frequencies in the resulting hybrid population can readily be predicted. Such calculations are made with the aid of formulae similar to those used for calculating the results of mixing solutions of different strengths. Conversely, if the Rh gene frequencies of a hybrid population are known, then the proportions of the parent populations from which they are derived can be calculated. For example, Glass has calculated that American Negroes represent the result of a cumulative admixture over many generations of approximately 30 per cent Caucasians. Similarly, Alvarez has shown that Dominicans are not merely a blend of Negroes and Caucasians, but also possess a small indigenous Amerindian component.

Atypical Rh-Hr types: This refers to human bloods which give reactions different from those characteristic of the "standard" Rh-Hr types. The most striking examples are the so-called types $\overline{\overline{Rh}}_0$ and Rh^w, which are characterized by the absence of both members of the pairs of factors rh'-hr' and rh''-hr''. Such individuals have been found to date in a few Caucasian families and in one Japanese family, and in almost every case have been the products of consanguineous marriages, as is to be expected with a gene of very low frequency. A number of variants of the phenotype Rh_0, notably Rh^V_0, $\mathfrak{R}h_0$, $\overline{Rh}_0$ and Rh_0 have been found among Negroes, as is to be expected from the high frequency of phenotype Rh_0 among Africans. An unusual Rh-Hr phenotype, rh, which apparently lacks all the known Rh-Hr factors, has been found in an Australian aborigene.

Rh types in chimpanzees: Among the infrahuman primates, chimpanzees have blood giving reactions with Rh-Hr and other blood grouping antisera most closely resembling those of human blood, as might be expected from their closer zoölogical relationship to man. The surface of the erythrocytes of chimpanzees apparently has the same number of loci for Rh-Hr agglutinogens as human red blood cells, since chimpanzee and human red cells maximally coated with Rh-Hr antibodies react to the same titer with anti-human globulin rabbit serum. The blood cells of all chimpanzees tested to date have given identical reactions, showing the presence of factors Rh_0 and

TABLE 22.—*Rh Gene Frequencies in Various Human Populations*

Populations	Investigators	Number of Persons Tested	Calculated Frequencies (%) of Genes						
			r	r'	r''	R^0	R^1	R^2	R^z
Caucasoids									
U.S.A.	Wiener et al.	2,390	36.65	1.23	0.52	3.73	42.70	15.06	0.05
U.S.A.	Unger et al.	7,317	38.3	1.4	0.8	2.8	42.1	15.1	—
England	Race et al.	2,000	38.86	0.98	1.19	2.57	42.05	14.11	0.24
Canada	Chown et al.	3,100	39.55	1.24	0.73	1.91	43.48	12.87	0.22
Spain	Race et al.	223	36.95	0	0.61	0.61	50.11	12.16	0.45
Czechoslovakia	Raska et al.	181	40.02	0.69	0.69	1.36	39.59	16.90	0.75
Basques	Chalmers et al.	383	53.16	1.47	0.25	0.50	37.56	7.07	0
Negroids, N.Y.C.	Wiener et al.	223	24.4	2.7	0	42.1	11.7	14.4	0
	Wiener et al.	200	27.39	0.89	0.89	43.32	17.30	9.02	0
Pygmies, Belgian Congo	Hubinont and Snoeck	94	10.5	0	0	63.2	6.2	19.5	0
Siamese	Phansanboom et al.	213	0	0	0	11.13	75.54	11.13	2.16
Papuans	Simmons and Graydon	100	0	0	0	2.1	94.3	2.0	1.6
Australian aborigines	Simmons and Graydon	234	0	12.87	0	8.54	56.42	20.09	2.08
New Caledonians	Simmons et al.	325	0	0	0	5.48	83.32	10.77	0.43
Mexican Indians	Wiener et al.	98	0	0	0	5.8	64.1	26.8	3.3
Navaho Indians	Boyd and Boyd	305	0	17.31	2.02	8.37	31.05	35.33	5.7

hr′, but the absence of rh′, as well as both members of the pair rh″ and hr″. All of the associated factors, Rh^A, Rh^B, Rh^C and Rh^D, are present, but the titers with the corresponding antisera are lower than those of typical human Rh-positive red cells, except for the blood factor Rh^C. For these reasons chimpanzee blood has been assigned the distinctive Rh-Hr phenotype symbol $(\overline{Rh}_0)^{Ch}$.

CHAPTER VIII
Medicolegal Applications

Disputed parentage: Like the A-B-O and M-N tests, Rh-Hr tests can be used to resolve certain problems of disputed parentage. Blood tests can be used only to disprove parentage and cannot be used to establish parentage. The reason for this is obvious since, if the blood of the putative parents match with that of the child in conformity with the genetic theory, this could be coincidental, while if the blood types do not match, parentage is excluded beyond doubt. Blood tests have therefore found their most frequent medicolegal application in cases of disputed paternity, where a man who is accused of the paternity of a baby born out of wedlock denies the charge. They have also found application in divorce and annulment proceedings, problems of interchange of babies in hospitals, kidnapping cases, inheritance disputes, and in immigration cases claiming derivative citizenship. Table 23 lists some of the authors' cases which illustrate the application of blood tests in parentage disputes.

Laws of heredity: When applying the Rh-Hr tests in cases of disputed parentage, the following laws of heredity are convenient to use. 1) The blood factors **Rh₀, rh′, rh″, hr′, hr″** and **rh^w** cannot appear in the blood of a child unless present in the blood of one or both parents. 2) A parent who is **rh′** negative cannot have a child who is **hr′** negative, and a parent who is **hr′** negative cannot have a child who is **rh′** negative. This law is based on the reciprocal relationship between the factor **rh′** and **hr′**, and is analogous to the law that the parent-child combinations type M parent—type N child and type N parent—type M child cannot occur. The discovery by Race and others of the existence of very rare Caucasians lacking both factors **rh′** and **hr′** makes necessary a very mild qualification when applying this law in medicolegal cases. 3) A parent who is **rh″** negative cannot have a child who is **hr″** negative, and a parent who is **hr″** negative cannot have a child who is **rh″** negative. To this law the same mild qualification must be made as to the second law, since rare individuals have been found, especially among Negroes, who lack both factors **rh″** and **hr″** (Wiener), in addition to the previously mentioned rare

Caucasians, who, besides lacking factors **rh'** and **hr'**, also lack **rh''** and **hr''**. A more common situation, occurring among Negroes, involves the factor **hr**^{S}, which occurs in association with factor **hr''**, as described by M. S. Shapiro. If the antiserum used in the tests is actually of specificity anti-**hr**^{S} instead of anti-**hr''**, this could result in an erroneous exclusion of paternity.

Table of matings: Table 24 gives the phenotypes which cannot occur in a child for matings between parents of the 18 different Rh-Hr types, as determined by tests with antisera of specificities anti-**Rh**$_0$, anti-**rh'**, anti-**rh''**, anti-**hr'** and anti-**hr''**. This compact table actually represents 324 matings, and it was possible to compress these into a 9×9 table by utilizing the symmetry of the Rh-Hr types with respect to the **Rh**$_0$ factor, as well as the symmetry of the "standard" Rh-Hr genes which form two sets of four genes each, namely, r, r', r'', r^y and R^0, R^1, R^2, R^z. Use was also made in the table of code numbers, which do not constitute a new nomenclature, but are used merely for the sake of convenience and compactness. Actually the table does not cover every mating, since it cannot be used without modification unless one or both parents are **Rh**$_0$ positive. When both parents are **Rh**$_0$ negative, it must be borne in mind that no **Rh**$_0$-positive type can occur in the children.

The reader may find it a stimulating exercise to construct this table for himself. As an example, the mating coded 1×2 is worked out as follows:

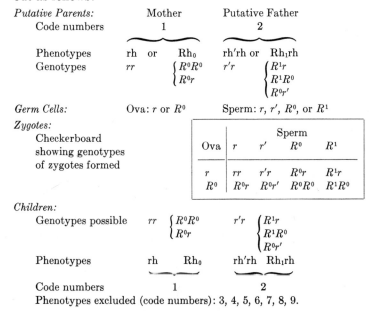

Putative Parents: Mother Putative Father
    Code numbers   1   2

Phenotypes   rh or Rh$_0$ rh'rh or Rh$_1$rh
Genotypes rr $\begin{cases} R^0R^0 \\ R^0r \end{cases}$ $r'r$ $\begin{cases} R^1r \\ R^1R^0 \\ R^0r' \end{cases}$

Germ Cells: Ova: r or R^0 Sperm: r, r', R^0, or R^1

Zygotes:
Checkerboard
showing genotypes
of zygotes formed

Ova	Sperm			
	r	r'	R^0	R^1
r	rr	$r'r$	R^0r	R^1r
R^0	R^0r	R^0r'	R^0R^0	R^1R^0

Children:
Genotypes possible rr $\begin{cases} R^0R^0 \\ R^0r \end{cases}$ $r'r$ $\begin{cases} R^1r \\ R^1R^0 \\ R^0r' \end{cases}$

Phenotypes   rh   Rh$_0$ rh'rh Rh$_1$rh

Code numbers   1   2
Phenotypes excluded (code numbers): 3, 4, 5, 6, 7, 8, 9.

TABLE 23.—*Application of Blood Tests in Disputed Parentage; Illustrative Cases*

	Putative Father	Mother	Children	Interpretation
1.	B MN kk Rh_1rh	B M kk Rh_1rh	A_1 MN kk Rh_1rh	Paternity excluded by A-B-O tests
2.	O MN kk rh	A_1 MN K rh	A_1 MN K rh	Findings inconclusive
3.	A_1 M kk Rh_1Rh_1	A_1 N kk Rh_1Rh_2	A_2 N K rh''	Paternity triply excluded by M-N, Rh-Hr, and Kell tests
4.	O M kk Rh_1Rh_2	O M kk Rh_1rh	A_1 MN kk Rh_1Rh_1	Paternity doubly excluded by A-B-O and M-N tests
5.*	O MN kk Rh_0	O MN kk Rh_0	O M kk Rh_0	Findings inconclusive
6.	B M Rh_1Rh_2	A_1 N Rh_1rh	O N Rh_1Rh_1	Paternity excluded by M-N tests
7.†	O MN kk Rh_1Rh_1	A_1 N kk Rh_2	O M kk Rh_1Rh_1	Maternity doubly excluded by M-N and Rh-Hr tests
8.	A_2 N Rh_1Rh_1	O N rh	A_1 MN rh	Paternity triply excluded by A_1-A_2, M-N, and Rh-Hr tests
9.	A_1 N rh'rh	A_1 N Rh_0	a) A_1 N Rh_0 b) O MN Rh_0	a) Findings inconclusive b) Paternity excluded by M-N tests for this child
10.	A_2 N rh	B MN Rh_2rh	A_2B N Rh_2rh	Findings inconclusive
11.	B N Rh_1Rh_1 kk ff	A_1 MN Rh_2rh kk ff	a) A_1 MN Rh_1rh kk ff b) O MN Rh_zRh_0 kk ff c) A_1 N Rh_zRh_0 kk ff	Findings inconclusive, that is, paternity not excluded for any of the three children
12.‡	O M Rh_1Rh_1	O MN Rh_2rh	O MN Rh_0	Paternity excluded by Rh-Hr tests
13.§	B N·ss rh P kk F	A_1 MN·S Rh_1Rh_1 P kk F	A_1B N·ss Rh_1rh P kk F	Findings inconclusive
14.	O MN·S Rh_zRh_0 pp kk F	A_1 N·ss Rh_2rh pp kk F	A_1 N·ss Rh_2rh pp kk F	Findings inconclusive

No.				Conclusion
15.	A_2 MN Rh_2Rh_2	O MN Rh_2Rh_2	A_1 MN Rh_zRh_0	Paternity doubly excluded by A_1–A_2 and **Rh-Hr** tests
16.*	A_1 MN Rh_0	O MN Rh_0	O MN Rh_0	Findings inconclusive
17.*	B MN Rh_1rh	O M Rh_1rh	A_2 MN Rh_0	Paternity excluded by the A-B-O tests
18.	O MN Rh_1Rh_1	O M rh	O MN rh'rh	Findings inconclusive
19.	O MN Rh_1Rh_1	B MN Rh_zRh_0	A_1B M Rh_2rh	Paternity excluded by A-B-O and **Rh-Hr** tests
20.	A_1 M rh	A_1 N Rh_1rh	A_1 MN Rh_zRh_0	Paternity excluded by the **Rh-Hr** tests
21.	A_1 M Rh_2rh	A_1 M Rh_1Rh_1	A_1 M Rh_zRh_1	Paternity excluded by the **Rh-Hr** tests
22.	O M Rh^wRh_1 kk	O MN Rh_1Rh_1 kk	O MN Rh_1Rh_1 kk	Findings inconclusive
23.	A_1 M Rh_1Rh_1 kk	O N Rh_1rh kk	a) A_2 MN Rh_1rh kk b) A_2 MN Rh_1Rh_1 kk c) A_2 MN Rh_1Rh_1 kk d) A_1 MN Rh_1rh kk e) A_1 MN Rh_1Rh_1 kk f) A_1 MN Rh_1rh kk	Paternity not excluded, and circumstantial evidence suggests that the accused man is the father, because all six children fit so perfectly with the genetic expectations

* Negroids.

† Chinese. After the Korean War many Chinese refugees tried to gain admittance to this country, claiming that their parents are American citizens. The immigration department uses blood tests routinely in such cases.

‡ East Indian. Here one must qualify one's conclusion slightly to allow for the rare agglutinogen lacking both the factors **rh'** and **hr'**.

§ Though listed in this table, the tests for the subgroups of A (A_1 and A_2), and the blood factors **S**, **rh**^{w}, **P**, **K**, and **F**, are not sufficiently reliable for routine medicolegal use. In unusual cases they may be tried, though they add little to the chances of excluding parentage, and the results should not be accepted at face value.

TABLE 24.—*Exclusion of Parentage by the Rh-Hr Blood Types*
(After Wiener: J. Forensic Med. May-June, 1962)

Phenotype of Putative Mother	Phenotype of Putative Father								
	1 rh Rh_0	2 rh'rh Rh_1rh	3 rh'rh' Rh_1Rh_1	4 rh''rh Rh_2rh	5 rh''rh'' Rh_2Rh_2	6 rh_2rh Rh_2Rh_0	7 rh_yrh' Rh_zRh_1	8 rh_yrh'' Rh_zRh_2	9 rh_yrh_y Rh_zRh_z
1 rh Rh_0	2, 3, 4, 5, 6, 7, 8, 9	3, 4, 5, 6, 7, 8, 9,	1, 3, 4, 5, 6, 7, 8, 9	2, 3, 5, 6, 7, 8, 9,	1, 2, 3, 5, 6, 7, 8, 9,	3, 5, 7, 8, 9	1, 3, 4, 5, 7, 8, 9	1, 2, 3, 5, 7, 8, 9	1, 2, 3, 4, 5, 7, 8, 9
2 rh'rh Rh_1rh	3, 4, 5, 6, 7, 8, 9	4, 5, 6, 7, 8, 9	1, 4, 5, 6, 7, 8, 9	3, 5, 7, 8, 9	1, 2, 3, 5, 7, 8, 9	5, 8, 9,	1, 4, 5, 8, 9	1, 2, 3, 5, 8, 9	1, 2, 3, 4, 5, 8, 9
3 rh'rh' Rh_1Rh_1	1, 3, 4, 5, 6, 7, 8, 9	1, 4, 5, 6, 7, 8, 9	1, 2, 4, 5, 6, 7, 8, 9	1, 3, 4, 5, 7, 8, 9	1, 2, 3, 4, 5, 7, 8, 9	1, 4, 5, 8, 9	1, 2, 4, 5, 6, 8, 9	1, 2, 3, 4, 5, 8, 9	1, 2, 3, 4, 5, 6, 8, 9
4 rh''rh Rh_2rh	2, 3, 5, 6, 7, 8, 9	3, 5, 7, 8, 9	1, 3, 4, 5, 7, 8, 9	2, 3, 6, 7, 8, 9	1, 2, 3, 6, 7, 8, 9	3, 7, 9	1, 3, 4, 5, 7, 9	1, 2, 3, 5, 7, 9	1, 2, 3, 4, 5, 7, 9
5 rh''rh'' Rh_2Rh_2	1, 2, 3, 5, 6, 7, 8, 9	1, 2, 3, 5, 7, 8, 9	1, 2, 3, 4, 5, 7, 8, 9	1, 2, 3, 6, 7, 8, 9	1, 2, 3, 4, 6, 7, 8, 9	1, 2, 3, 7, 9	1, 2, 3, 4, 5, 7, 9	1, 2, 3, 4, 6, 7, 9	1, 2, 3, 4, 5, 6, 7, 9

Code	Phenotypes	1	2	3	4	5	6	7	8	9
6	rh_y rh, Rh_z Rh_0	3, 5, 7, 8, 9	5, 8, 9	1, **4**, 5, 8, 9	3, 7, 9	1, 2, 3, 7, 9	None	1, **4**, 5	1, 2, 3	1, 2, 3, **4**, 5
7	rh_y rh', Rh_z Rh_1	1, 3, **4**, 5, 7, 8, 9	1, **4**, 5, 8, 9	1, 2, **4**, 5, **6**, 8, 9	1, 3, **4**, 5, 7, 9	1, 2, 3, **4**, 5, 7, 9	1, **4**, 5	1, 2, **4**, 5, **6**	1, 2, 3, **4**, 5	1, 2, 3, **4**, 5, **6**, 8
8	rh_y rh'', Rh_z Rh_2	1, 2, 3, 5, 7, 8, 9	1, 2, 3, 5, 8, 9	1, 2, 3, **4**, 5, 8, 9	1, 2, 3, 7, 9	1, 2, 3, **4**, **6**, 7, 9	1, 2, 3	1, 2, 3	1, 2, 3, **4**, **6**, 7	1, 2, 3, **4**, 5, **6**, 7
9	rh_y rh_y, Rh_z Rh_z	1, 2, 3, **4**, 5, 7, 8, 9	1, 2, 3, **4**, 5, 8, 9	1, 2, 3, **4**, 5, **6**, 8, 9	1, 2, 3, **4**, 5, 7, 9	1, 2, 3, **4**, 5, **6**, 7, 9	1, 2, 3, **4**, 5	1, 2, 3, **4**	1, 2, 3, **4**	1, 2, 3, **4**, 5, **6**, 7, 8

Bold face figures represent phenotypes of children for whom *maternity* is excluded.

This table is to be applied only to matings in which at least one of the parents is Rh_0 positive. Where both parents are Rh_0 negative, necessarily all Rh_0-positive children are excluded. For example, see text.

The phenotypes corresponding to the code numbers are given in the marginal headings; e.g., 1 is the code number for phenotypes rh and Rh_0.

Phenotypes Rh_ZRh_0 and rh_yrh and blood factor hr: The phenotype Rh_ZRh_0 which occurs in 14 to 15 per cent of Caucasians is defined as having all five factors, **Rh_0**, **rh′**, **rh″**, **hr′** and **hr″** (*cf.* table 10). Among Caucasians, six possible genotypes can occur according to the eight-allele theory, and these naturally fall into two sets depending on the presence or absence of the rare genes R^Z and r^y, as follows:

Set 1 (frequency 13.5 per cent): genotypes R^1R^2, $R^1r″$, and $R^2r′$

Set 2 (frequency 0.2 per cent): genotypes R^Zr, R^ZR^0, and R^0r^y

From the standpoint of medicolegal application, the importance of this subdivision is that a person who is in set 1 cannot have a child of type rh or type Rh_0, while a person who belongs in set 2 can. As can be seen, the odds that a person of the phenotype Rh_ZRh_0 belongs to set 1 rather than set 2 are about 67 to 1. For courtroom use, however, even such high odds do not constitute adequate evidence. With the aid of anti-**hr** serum the set to which an Rh_ZRh_0 person belongs can be determined, because this reagent reacts only with the cells of individuals carrying either gene R^0 or r. Thus, if the blood cells react negatively with anti-**hr** serum the individual belongs to set 1 (designated phenotype Rh_1Rh_2), while if his blood reacts positively he belongs to set 2 (designated Rh_Zrh). Similarly, the exact genotype of an individual of the rare phenotype rh_yrh (*cf.* table 10) can be determined by tests with anti-hr serum as follows: **hr** positive = genotype r^yr, and **hr** negative = genotype $r′r″$. The reagent anti-**hr** is rare and difficult to obtain, but it is fortunately possible to conserve the small quantities available since the preliminary tests with the "standard" reagents will indicate in which cases tests for the factor **hr** are likely to yield useful information. A few illustrative cases are shown in table 25.

Chances of excluding paternity: The chances that a man falsely accused of paternity can be excluded by a blood test. This varies with the distribution of the types in the population; e.g., if everyone belonged to the same blood type the tests would be entirely worthless for the purpose. Among Caucasians the chances of excluding paternity are close to 20 per cent for the A-B-O groups, about 18 per cent for the three M-N types, and about 25 per cent for the Rh-Hr types (tests for the factors **Rh_0**, **rh′**, **rh″**, **hr′** and **hr″**). The combined chances of excluding paternity when tests for all three systems are

TABLE 25.—*Cases Illustrating the Medicolegal Application of* **hr** *Tests in Disputed Paternity*

Case No.*	Blood of	Rh-Hr Type	hr Factor	Phenotype or Genotype	Comment
1	Putative father	Rh_zRh_0	−	Rh_1Rh_2	Paternity
	Mother	Rh_zRh_0	−	Rh_1Rh_2	excluded
	Child	Rh_2rh	+		
2	Putative father	Rh_1Rh_1	−		Paternity
	Mother	Rh_zRh_0	+	Rh_zrh	not excluded
	Child	Rh_1rh	+		
3†	Putative father	Rh_zRh_0	−	Rh_1Rh_2	Paternity
	Mother	rh	+		excluded
	Child	rh	+		
4	Putative father	Rh_1Rh_1	−		Paternity
	Mother	rh_yrh	+	$r^y r$	not excluded
	Child	Rh_1rh	+		
5‡	Putative father	Rh_zRh_0	+	Rh_zrh	Paternity
	Mother	rh	+		not excluded
	Child	Rh_zRh_0	+	Rh_zrh	

* In the cases listed here, tests for the A-B-O groups and the M-N types gave inconclusive results.

† In this case the mother's blood is not needed to exclude paternity.

‡ From Dunsford et al. Here the blood tests not only failed to exclude, but instead provided circumstantial evidence that the man was actually the father, in view of the rare Rh-Hr type involved.

carried out are not merely the sum of these because the results of tests can overlap, and doubly or triply exclude the same putative father. The true combined chances are somewhat above 50 per cent, as can be calculated with the aid of the formula:

$$P = 1 - (1 - P_1)(1 - P_2)(1 - P_3) \ldots (1 - P_n)$$

where P_1, P_2, P_3 . . . P_n are the respective chances of excluding paternity by independent tests. Obviously, it becomes more and more difficult to increase the chances of exclusion, and the ideal of 100 per cent can never be reached, no matter how many different tests are used.

The newer blood factors: During the past decade many new blood factors have been discovered (*cf.* table 20). Most of these have not been studied intensively enough, however, for medicolegal application, and sera of satisfactory avidity and specificity are difficult and sometimes impossible to obtain. For results that are at all reproducible the delicate and sometimes elaborate tests must be carried out most painstakingly and, above all, objectively (blind test). Since the combined use of all these new blood factors raises the chances of excluding paternity by only 10 to 15 per cent, they may not be worth the additional effort and expense entailed. Besides, an erroneous exclusion of parentage that could easily result when the newer tests are used might serve to discredit the valuable A-B-O, M-N, and Rh-Hr tests in the eyes of the court.

Circumstantial evidence of paternity: In rare cases the blood tests provide circumstantial evidence of parentage, namely, when the same rare blood type is present in the child and in the putative parent. For example, when the mother belongs to type rh, while the baby and the putative father both belong to type rh', or type rh'', or type Rh_1^w, etc., the evidence would strongly suggest that the accused man actually is the father, though one must still bear in mind the possibility of coincidence.

Exclusion of maternity: Blood tests have been used successfully to solve problems of disputed maternity (*cf.* case 7, table 23). Maternity is excluded if any of the following mother-child combinations are encountered: mother O—child AB; mother AB—child O; mother M—child N; mother N—child M; mother **rh'** negative—child **hr'** negative; mother **hr'** negative—child **rh'** negative. The following may be used only as circumstantial evidence of nonmaternity: mother A_1B—child A_2; mother A_2—child A_1B; mother **rh''** negative—child **hr''** negative; mother **hr''** negative—child **rh''** negative; mother Rh_1Rh_2—child rh or Rh_0; mother rh or Rh_0—child Rh_1Rh_2.

Index